# HPV: THE HUMAN PAPILLOMAVIRUS
## PATIENT ADVOCATE

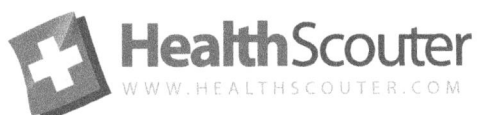

HealthScouter.com - Equity Press
5055 Canyon Crest Drive
Riverside, California 92507

www.healthscouter.com

Purchasing this book entitles you to free updates at www.healthscouter.com/HPV

Edited By: Shana McKibbin

Includes HPV from Wikipedia http://en.wikipedia.org/wiki/HPV
Includes HPV Vaccine from Wikipedia http://en.wikipedia.org/wiki/HPV_vaccine

HealthScouter HPV: Understanding HPV Testing: The Human Papillomavirus Patient Advocate (HealthScouter HPV)

ISBN 978-1-60332-094-8

Edited components are copyright ©2009 Equity Press and HealthScouter all rights reserved.

Permission is granted to copy, distribute, and/or modify this document under the terms of the GNU Free Documentation License, Version 1.2 or any later version published by the Free Software Foundation; with no Invariant Sections, no Front-Cover Texts, and no Back-Cover Texts. A copy of the license is included in the section entitled "GNU Free Documentation License."

**Trademarks:** All trademarks are the property of their respective owners. Equity Press is not associated with any product or vendor mentioned in this book.

**Important**

**NEVER DISREGARD PROFESSIONAL MEDICAL ADVICE, OR DELAY SEEKING IT, BECAUSE OF SOMETHING YOU HAVE READ IN THIS BOOK. ALWAYS SEEK PROFESSIONAL MEDICAL ADVICE BEFORE ACTING UPON INFORMATION READ IN THIS BOOK.**

HealthScouter and Equity Press do not provide medical advice. The contents of this book are for informational purposes only and are not intended to substitute for professional medical advice, diagnosis or treatment. Always seek advice from a qualified physician or health care professional about any medical concern, and do not disregard professional medical advice because of anything you may read in this book or on a HealthScouter Web site. The views of individuals quoted in this book are not necessarily those of HealthScouter or Equity Press.

While this book is intended to be a medium for the exchange of information and ideas, it is not meant in any way to be a substitute for sound medical advice; neither should it be viewed as a trusted source of such advice. The views expressed in these messages are not those of any qualified medical association, and the publisher is not responsible for the validity of the information communicated herein or for consequences that may arise from acting upon this information. The publisher is not responsible for any content found in the book that may be deemed offensive, inappropriate, inaccurate or medically unsound. The information you find here is only for the purpose of discussion and should not be the basis for any medical decision. The content is not intended to be a substitute for professional medical advice, diagnosis or treatment.

The information presented is not to be considered complete, nor does it contain all medical resource information that may be relevant, and therefore it is not intended to be a substitute for seeking medical treatment and/or appropriate care.

By reading this book and parts of the Web site, you agree under all circumstances to hold harmless, and to refrain from seeking remedy from, the owners of this book. The publisher shall disclaim all liability to you for damages, costs or expenses, including legal and medical fees, related to your reliance on anything derived from this book or Web site or its contents. Furthermore, Equity Press assumes no liability for any and all claims arising out of the said use, regardless of the cause, effects, or fault.

Equity Press and HealthScouter do not endorse any company or product, and listing on the HealthScouter Web site is not linked to corporate sponsorship. We do not make a claim to being comprehensive or up to date. If you would like to recommend information to include in this book, please contact us – we would be very happy to hear from you.

Purchasing this book entitles you to free updates as they are available. Please register your book at www.healthscouter.com

# TABLE OF CONTENTS

Introduction and Motivation .................................................. 6

How to Use This Book .......................................................... 12

Introduction to HPV ........................................................... 15

Prevalence .................................................................... 25
    United States ............................................................ 25

Cervical Cancer ............................................................... 31

HPV Lifecycle ................................................................. 35
    Latency Period ........................................................... 36

HPV Types and Associated Diseases ............................................. 37

Cancer ........................................................................ 39

Warts ......................................................................... 43
    Skin Warts ............................................................... 43
    Genital Warts ............................................................ 44

Respiratory Papillomatosis .................................................... 49

HPV in Immunocompromised Patients ............................................. 51

Cervical Cancer Prevention .................................................... 53
    Pap Smear Screening ...................................................... 53

HPV Testing ................................................................... 69

HPV Testing in Males .......................................................... 73

HPV Vaccines .................................................................. 77

Condoms ....................................................................... 85

Microbicides .................................................................. 87

Treatment ..................................................................... 89

HPV Vaccine ................................................................... 91

History of Vaccine ............................................................ 113
    Therapeutic HPV Vaccines ................................................. 113

Epidemiology.................................................................115
    Cutaneous HPVs........................................................115
    Genital HPVs .........................................................116

Perinatal Transmission ........................................................117

History of Discovering a Link Between HPV and Cancer ............................119

References – HPV .............................................................124

References – HPV Vaccine .....................................................130

GNU Free Documentation License ................................................136

Index ........................................................................144

**HEALTH**SCOUTER

## INTRODUCTION AND MOTIVATION

Dear Reader,

I like to think of myself as a polite, well-reasoned person. I rarely speak out or complain. When a waitress spills something on me, or if my meal is cold—or if I'm overcharged—I generally try to be as polite as possible. I don't like to make very many waves. I often secretly hope that the manager will hear about my predicament and come out and offer me a free meal, or something similar. I generally hope that my polite and respectful demeanor pays off. And it does happen from time to time. You know, I think many people are brought up to believe that this is just good manners. It's how you're supposed to behave. And if you knew me personally, I think you'd agree that I'm generally pretty reserved. Of course my wife may raise an objection or two (!), but I really believe that it's important to treat others as you would like to be treated. We're talking about the golden rule here—it works well and it applies to almost every life circumstance.

But I have to admit that when it comes to my health, or the health of someone I care about—all bets are off. I want to know what's going on—when, why, where, and how. And I make these feelings known. I tend to get downright assertive. It's just something I feel very strongly about. And I feel that when you are in a hospital, or if you're brushing up against the healthcare system, that you should feel the same way. It's unfamiliar turf, and the professionals who work in this system often take advantage of their positions. They may use some jargon to hide the whole truth—or they may say something without checking to make sure you understand completely. They may present the options that are best for them, perhaps the most profitable or convenient. Now I'm not saying this goes on everywhere. There are many professionals in the business of health who go out of their way to make sure you have the best care. And I'm not suggesting that you should become a bully, or purposefully annoying—absolutely not. But I am suggesting that I think it's OK for you to step outside of your typical comfort zone, and put on your patient advocate hat. Because you, the patient or patient advocate, care the most about your care—not the medical system or healthcare providers.

HealthScouter was created to help patients become better advocates for their own medical care. Because when it comes to your healthcare, the stakes are high. There are none higher. And healthcare is one area where consumers (us, the sick people) are notoriously unaware of their options. And that's why I'm publishing these books. To help you understand your options, and to help you get the best care possible. I want to help you become a better advocate for yourself and for your loved ones.

It's my sincere hope that you can take this book with you to the hospital, to be read in the waiting room or by the bedside—and when you see a relevant patient comment you can use this book to ask questions of your health care providers. My advice: Ask lots of questions! Providers are busy people who generally go about their business with little questioning, delivering care as they see fit—making quick decisions—and again, nobody is going to care as much about your health as you. So now, more than ever, you need tools at your disposal to get the best care possible. One of the tools at your disposal is this HealthScouter book and the material within. You need to be armed with questions, and you need to ask questions all of the time. And so the difficult part is now to understand the right questions to ask.

That brings me to an explanation of how these books are structured. HealthScouter books include a number of what we call patient comments. These patient comments are summaries of what people have experienced. They're first hand accounts of what you may expect. These experiences effectively help you "catch up," and understand what outcomes are possible. They expose you to the treatments are available, and provide insight as to potential outcomes. They help you understand what other people are doing. So if you find yourself stuck feeling like you're receiving substandard medical care—or if you need a push to broach the subject, you can take this book to your provider and say, "Hey, I read here that another patient had this treatment—is that an option for me? If not, Why?" I believe that other peoples' experience is the most valuable way for you to formulate and build a list of good questions for your healthcare providers.

That notion is at the core of the HealthScouter philosophy.

So HealthScouter, by providing patient comments about a particular medical condition, will help expose you to what other people have experienced about a particular medical problem. If you know what other people have experienced, you can better understand what your options are. You'll be better informed and you'll have some questions to ask—it'll be like you've had access to dozens of other people who have gone through the same thing you're going through. And so armed, maybe you'll be able to move through your condition and get back on the road to health, and maybe you'll be able to do this with more grace than I have. And that is my sincere wish.

It's also my wish that perhaps when a doctor or nurse sees this little blue book, that they'll think twice about the care they're about to provide—knowing that the owner is a little bit better prepared, a little bit better armed—and yes, maybe even downright assertive.

I hope this book helps.

Yours truly,

Jim Stewart

San Diego, California

# HPV: THE HUMAN PAPILLOMAVIRUS

# HEALTHSCOUTER

## HOW TO USE THIS BOOK

The purpose of HealthScouter is to help you understand your medical condition as quickly and easily as possible. We believe this can best be accomplished by reading about other people and their experiences negotiating their health and care. We try to leave out complicated medical jargon. And we've spent a considerable amount of time structuring this book so that it's easy to use. It's important to know that this is not the sort of book you read from beginning to end. Of course you may do so, but this book is more meaningful if you flip through quickly and scan for applicable material. Again, it's all about the patient commentary: The darkly shaded comments ▮ indicate one patient initiating a new discussion, and the light or clear comments 🗩 are other comments associated with that same condition. So you should begin by looking for information from other patients who are experiencing the same aspect of the same medical condition that you studying. You can do this quickly by scanning through the book, focusing on the dark shaded comment boxes. By scanning the patient comments you'll find information about various aspects of a condition, all grouped together, in an easy-to-read format. In this way you can immediately begin reading about other patients and their experiences with your particular medical condition – and you can benefit immediately from their experiences.

## INTRODUCTION TO HPV

A human papillomavirus (HPV) is a papillomavirus that infects the skin and mucous membranes of humans. It impacts the health of women far more than it impacts men. Approximately 130 HPV types have been identified. Some HPV types can cause warts (verrucae) or some types of cancer, while others have no symptoms. "Most people who become infected with HPV do not even know they have it."[1]

About 30–40 HPV types are typically transmitted through sexual contact and infect the anogenital region. Some sexually transmitted HPV types may cause genital warts. Persistent infection with "high-risk" HPV types — different from the ones that cause warts — may progress to precancerous lesions and invasive cancer. HPV infection is a cause of nearly all cases of cervical cancer.[2] However most infections with these types do not cause disease.

A cervical Pap smear is used to detect cellular abnormalities. This allows targeted surgical removal of condylomatous and/or potentially precancerous lesions prior to the development of invasive cervical cancer. Although the widespread use of Pap testing has reduced the incidence and lethality of cervical cancer in developed countries, the disease still kills several hundred thousand women per year worldwide.[3] HPV vaccines, Gardasil and Cervarix, which prevent infection with some of the sexually transmitted HPV types that cause the most disease may lead to further decreases in the incidence of HPV-induced cancers.[4]

*Human papillomavirus (HPV) is the name of a group of viruses that infect the skin. There are more than 70 different types of HPV. Certain types of HPV cause warts on the hands or feet, and other types can cause warts on the genitals. But some people never have warts they can see and many never get warts, so most people with HPV do not know they have it. About 30 of these types are sexually transmitted and cause genital HPV. Some types of genital HPV may cause genital warts, while other types of genital HPV are linked to abnormal cell changes on the cervix (detected through Pap smears).*

*Genital HPV is passed by skin-to-skin and genital contact, primarily during vaginal and anal intercourse. It might also be possible to pass it during oral sex.*

*I've got a lot of these very small flesh-colored/whitish bumps on well multiple areas of the*

# HPV: THE HUMAN PAPILLOMAVIRUS

vagina. They don't hurt but I'm concerned that it may be something (I've had these for as long as I can remember). Are these normal or should I go see my doctor?

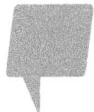

I am a little confused about HPV. My girlfriend has had abnormal Pap smears for the last 2 years and recently the doctor did further testing and told her she has polyps. Now she did not say anything to my about having HPV or that what she has is sexually transmitted or anything. However recently I noticed dots on the base of my penis, shaft, and head that I am beginning to think are warts. Is it possible if she has HPV on her cervix/uterus that I could get HPV in the warts form? Also assuming that are warts on my penis will they go away on their own in time?

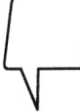

Yep it is most likely that it is HPV. The thing about the disease is most people do not know about it. I am not sure if she knew that she had it or not or realized that it is very contagious... that is not for me to decipher. Anyways you should go get check because the quicker you get in for treatment the sooner your body will build immunity to it and become clear of it.

17

# HEALTHSCOUTER

> I realize the virus never goes away and I know HPV is short for human papillomavirus virus. But doesn't your body build natural immunity to warts and they go away over time? I have had these bumps probably two weeks and they are not noticeable unless I am in bright lighting, or after I have sex they turn red. They are very small so I figure if I just let them go they will go away eventually right? Also can I spread them to other parts of my body by touching them? Or shaving the area can that spread them more down there?

> I would say it is very likely you have the warts and, NO, they will not go away on their own. You need to see a doctor ASAP.

> I had sex a few weeks ago. I am due for my Pap smear this month. If I have been infected, will the smear test show it now or I have to wait for the virus to start working. How quickly can the changes be detected since the last sexual contact?

> Warts typically show up between 2–8 weeks later, but I haven't read any specific timeline for cervical cell changes. Since they are part of the same virus family, and some of the wart strains can also cause cervical cell changes, the timeline might be similar.

# HPV: THE HUMAN PAPILLOMAVIRUS

 *How soon can I get tested for HPV after I believe I have been exposed to it?*

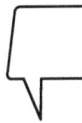 I don't know many places that do tests for HPV, or if there is a test or not. I got it checked out when I started showing symptoms. Be sure to get a Pap smear every year to check for abnormal cells. HPV isn't always symptomatic.

 *If you and your partner are both virgins is there still a chance of catching a STD when not using a condom??? I don't know if this sounds silly or not but I was just thinking that STD's have to start somewhere so couldn't they be in someone's body all along?*

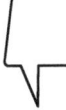 The only way to get an STD is having sex with someone who is affected with it. The other person got the disease from someone else who was infected with it and so on. The only exception to this is from your mom - certain things (like AIDS) can be passed from mother to child. But I'd say if you both are 100% true virgins (including oral), there is almost no way either one of you could get an STD from each other.

By the way, you can catch HPV, even while using a condom.

> I know this sounds gross, but I need to know if I should get checked for HPV on my butt if I have and have had anal sex. Lately, my anus has been really sore and itchy, sometimes bloody?

That sounds like it needs to be checked out by a doctor regardless of whether or not it's HPV. I know low-risk HPV can show up in your anus; I'm not sure if it could be high-risk.

HPV does not make you sore, itchy, or bloody. If you have warts, they may cause some problems, but you would see or feel them and it would be obvious they were the cause.

You might have some other sort of infection there, if the anal passage was torn during intercourse.

By the way, condoms are only minimally effective in preventing HPV transmission.

> Can you have sex when you have HPV?

Yes, though as with any STD, you should let your partner know so that he or she can make an informed decision.

# HPV: THE HUMAN PAPILLOMAVIRUS

 *Does HPV cause blood in your urine? If so what does it mean?*

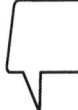 I cannot think of any reason for HPV to cause your urine to have blood in it. It sounds like a bladder or kidney infection. Please get to the doctor today!

 *How do I ensure my sexual partner doesn't get HPV?*

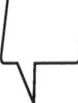 You cannot necessarily prevent your partner from getting HPV. You can reduce the risks through the use of condoms but HPV is transmitted through skin to skin contact. This includes the skin and mucous membranes which includes through oral sex. HPV can be contracted without ever having intercourse. Often it is transmitted because the skin surrounding the unprotected condom is infected. Since there is no test for men, and they usually show no symptoms, they pass it along without ever knowing it. Even if she shows up with it a month from now does not necessarily mean she got it from you. It is almost impossible to determine from whom a woman contracts HPV because it can be dormant for months or years so unless she had absolutely no genital contact with anyone else you cannot specifically pinpoint one individual as having given it to you. If your partner is under 26,

I would suggest she get the Gardasil vaccine which can help protect again the four major types of HPV (two low risk and two high risk).

Are men the ones that infect women with the HPV virus?

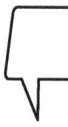
People are infected by their partners, male or female. So a heterosexual woman would be infected by a male, and a heterosexual male would be infected by a female.

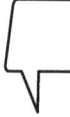
Having many partners does increase the likelihood of getting HPV, but there are other factors as well. You can be in good health, but still get it. Not always from sex, as far as I know. Yes, men can have it too. It is very contagious.

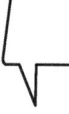
It is very rare to get HPV without having sex. I would still do everything I could to prevent this, to be safe and healthy, even if you are not having sex.

How can a person who hasn't had sex or any type of contact with anyone get HPV? We are very confused. We are thinking of repeating the test in another hospital.

# HPV: THE HUMAN PAPILLOMAVIRUS

*A very valid question. The hospital told my wife that she is HPV positive but we are both sure that no sexual relationships occurred before our marriage.*

There are three possibilities: a) hospital lab is wrong; b) there is other way to get it other than sexual; c) inherited from a parent.

I think it is physically impossible to 'never have any type of contact with anyone'.

There are also more strains of non-genital HPV than there are of genital HPV, so if you mean getting it with no sexual contact, then yes, there are still lots of strains of HPV you can get w/o sexual contact.

Just look at all the kids with warts on their hands or feet. I seriously doubt they got it through sexual contact.

**HEALTH**SCOUTER

# PREVALENCE

## United States

HPV is estimated to be the most common sexually transmitted infection in the United States.[5] Most sexually active men and women will probably acquire genital HPV infection at some point in their lives.[6] The American Social Health Association reported estimates that about 75–80% of sexually active Americans will be infected with HPV at some point in their lifetime.[7][8] By the age of 50 more than 80% of American women will have contracted at least one strain of genital HPV.[9][10][11]

It was estimated that in the year 2000, there were approximately 6.2 million new HPV infections among Americans aged 15–44; of these, an estimated 74% occurred to people between ages 15–24.[12] Of the STDs studied, genital HPV was the most commonly acquired.[12]

Estimates of HPV prevalence vary from 14% to more than 90%.[13] One reason for the difference is that some studies report women who currently have a detectable infection, while other studies report women who have ever had a detectable infection.[14][15]

Another cause of discrepancy is the difference in strains that were tested for.

One study found that, during 2003–2004, at any given time, 26.8% of women aged 14 to 59 were infected with at least one type of HPV. This was higher than previous estimates. 15.2% were infected with one or more of the high-risk types that can cause cancer. However only 3.4% were infected with one or more of the four types prevented by the Gardasil vaccine, which was lower than previous estimates.[5][16]

| HPV prevalence by age[5] ||
| --- | --- |
| Age (years) | Prevalence (%) |
| 14 to 19 | 24.5% |
| 20 to 24 | 44.8% |
| 25 to 29 | 27.4% |
| 30 to 39 | 27.5% |
| 40 to 49 | 25.2% |
| 50 to 59 | 19.6% |
| 14 to 59 | 26.8% |

Note that prevalence decreases with age. This may be due to HPV infection being cleared by the immune system, or sinking to undetectable levels while still present in the body. HPV will probably remain in the infected person's cells for an indefinite time--most often in a latent state, but occasionally producing symptoms or disease. Recent studies from the Albert Einstein College of Medicine and from the University of Washington suggest that HPV may eventually be cleared in most people with well functioning immune systems. It appears that in some cases the virus does remain in the body indefinitely, producing symptoms if the immune system weakens.

*Most people do not know they have HPV (even one or many strains). For that reason, if a person has more than one sexual partner in his/her lifetime, it is very likely he/she has contracted at least one strain of HPV. Because most people do not know they have HPV, if they change partners, then they are spreading any strain of HPV he/she might have, as well as being exposed to (possibly) new strains.*

*Can a married couple be tested for the virus, and if clean, can any one of them catch it if they only are with each other? Or is the virus just around like the cold virus, and you can catch it in some other way than sexual contact?*

*HPV is spread by skin to skin contact. The 20+ (out of 100+) strains of HPV that effect the genitals*

(vulva, vagina, penis, anus, rectum, mouth/throat) are spread by skin to skin contact with other genitals. If there has been any skin to skin contact (even without sexual intercourse) then it is possible to spread HPV.

Something like 80% of women, by the time they are 50 (and assuming they had some sort of sexual contact in their life time) have been exposed to at least one strain of HPV. It is VERY common. The good news is that most people are able to "fight" the virus so it doesn't cause any problems. It doesn't go away, it stays in the body, but it doesn't cause problems.

Of those 20+ strains that affect the genitals, they are divided into 2 parts: low risk and high risk. Low risk cause warts, high risk cause changes that can result in cancer (of the various body parts already mentioned). Low risk doesn't cause cancer, high risk doesn't cause warts.

Testing: There is a HPV/DNA test that a doctor can use on a woman when she has her annual pap. Most doctors do not do the test on women under 30 because they are very likely to fight the virus into not causing damage. There is a test, but from what I understand it is used rarely - very rarely.

# HPV: THE HUMAN PAPILLOMAVIRUS

> What ethnic group most likely to suffer from HPV?

> I have never read any research on this. I recommend searching the Center for Disease Control's website for this type of research information.

> This is an odd question. Since HPV is a virus, not genetic, it's like asking ethnic group is most likely to get the flu.

**HEALTH**SCOUTER

## CERVICAL CANCER

Women who do not have regular cervical cancer screenings substantially increase their risk of developing cancer[3], because potentially precancerous lesions are not detected and they do not receive appropriate follow-up.[17] An estimated 11% of American women do not have regular cervical cancer screenings.[3] The American Cancer Society estimates that in 2008, about 11,070 women in the United States will be diagnosed with invasive cervical cancer, and about 3,870 US women will die from this disease.[18]

*I have just found out that an ex girlfriend has been diagnosed with cervical cancer, is this something I should be worried about? Do I need to see my doctor?*

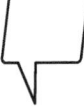
*You mean did you catch cancer from her? No. It's possible you gave her (or she gave you) HPV, human papillomavirus (aka genital warts), which is the leading cause of cervical cancer and is an STD. Wouldn't hurt to get checked, men are often asymptomatic- which is why it's more likely you gave it to her than she to you.*

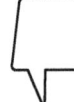
*Do you know if you have HPV? Not many tests for males. Ever had any cauliflower sores in the pubic*

area or buttocks. If so then you may have given her HPV which leads to cervical cancer in women.

HPV is the leading cause of penile cancer in males, as well.

If there any lumps or odd spots which don't heal develop, I would get them looked at quickly.

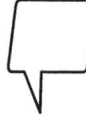Cervical cancer is caused by certain strains of HPV. You can't catch cervical cancer from her but if you've been having sex with her, you can be pretty sure you have whatever strain(s) of HPV she has. And as tommy124 points out, HPV can cause penile cancer. It also causes oral and throat cancer but all these forms are very rare.

Also should point out that the logic that it is more likely you gave it to her makes no sense, unless she was a virgin and you were her only partner. It is just as likely she got it from a previous or later boyfriend. First off, all men are asymptomatic for the strains that cause cervical cancer (unless they themselves have cancer) because the strains that cause cancer are not the strains that cause warts

You can't tell or assume who gave the HPV to whom, and is a waste of time to try and guess. The only thing you can be sure of is that you have been *exposed to at least one strain of HPV that causes cervical cancer and you should be concerned that any partners you've had after that are good about keeping up with their Pap tests (something all sexually active women should do).*

## HPV LIFECYCLE

The HPV lifecycle strictly follows the differentiation program of the host keratinocyte. It is thought that the HPV virion infects epithelial tissues through micro-abrasions, whereby the virion associates with putative receptors such as alpha integrins and laminins, leading to entry of the virions into basal epithelial cells through clathrin-mediated endocytosis and/or caveolin-mediated endocytosis depending on the type of HPV. At this point, the viral genome is transported to the nucleus by unknown mechanisms and establishes itself at a copy number between 10–200 viral genomes per cell. A sophisticated transcriptional cascade then occurs as the host keratinocyte begins to divide and become increasingly differentiated in the upper layers of the epithelium. The viral oncogenes, E6 and E7, are thought to modify the cell cycle so as to retain the differentiating host keratinocyte in a state that is amiable to the amplification of viral genome replication and consequent late gene expression. E6 in association with host E6 AP (associated protein), which has ubiquitin ligase activity act to ubiquitinate p53 leading to its proteosomal degradation. E7 (inoncogenic HPV's) acts as the primary transforming protein. E7 competes for pRb binding, freeing the transcription factor E2F to transactivate its targets, thus pushing the cell cycle forwards. All HPV can induce transient proliferation, but only 16 and 18 can immortalise cell intes (in vitro). It has also been shown that HPV 16 and 18 cannot immortalise primary rat cells alone, there needs to be activation of the ras oncogene. In the upper layers of the host epithelium, the late genes L1 and L2 are transcribed/translated and serve as structural proteins which encapsidate (Encapsidation is the process of incorporating a nucleic acid sequence (e.g., a vector, or a viral genome) into a viral particle) the amplified viral genomes. Virions can then be sloughed off in the dead squames of the host epithelium and the viral lifecycle continues.[19]

## Latency Period

Once an HPV viron invades a cell, an active infection occurs, and the virus can be transmitted. Several months to years may elapse before squamous intraepithelial lesions (SIL) develop and can be clinically detected. The time from active infection to clinically detectable disease makes it difficult for someone who has become infected to establish which partner was the source of infection.

# HPV: THE HUMAN PAPILLOMAVIRUS

## HPV TYPES AND ASSOCIATED DISEASES

*Notable HPV types and associated diseases*

Over 100 different HPV types have been identified and are referred to by number. Types 16, 18, 31, 33, 35, 39, 45, 51, 52, 56, 58, 59, and 68 are "high-risk" sexually transmitted HPVs and may lead to the development of cervical intraepithelial neoplasia (CIN), vulvar intraepithelial neoplasia (VIN), penile intraepithelial neoplasia (PIN), and/or anal intraepithelial neoplasia (AIN).

| Disease | HPV type |
|---|---|
| Common warts | 2, 7 |
| Plantar warts | 1, 2, 4 |
| Flat warts | 3, 10 |
| Anogenital warts | 6, 11, 42, 43, 44, 55 and others |
| Genital cancers | 16, 18, 31, 33, 35, 39, 45, 51, 52, 56, 58, 59, 68, 73, 82 |
| Epidermodysplasia verruciformis | more than 15 types |
| Focal epithelial hyperplasia (oral) | 13, 32 |
| Oral papillomas | 6, 7, 11, 16, 32 |

**HEALTH**SCOUTER

## CANCER

About a dozen HPV types (including types 16, 18, 31 and 45) are called "high-risk" types because they can lead to cervical cancer, as well as anal cancer, vulvar cancer, and penile cancer.[20] Several types of HPV, particularly type 16, have been found to be associated with oropharyngeal squamous-cell carcinoma, a form of head and neck cancer.[21] HPV-induced cancers often have viral sequences integrated into the cellular DNA. Some of the HPV "early" genes, such as E6 and E7, are known to act as oncogenes that promote tumor growth and malignant transformation.

The p53 protein prevents cell growth and stimulates apoptosis in the presence of DNA damage. It causes BAX protein upregulation, which blocks the anti-apoptotic effects of the mitochondrial BCL-2 protein. In addition, p53 also upregulates the p21 protein, which blocks the formation of the Cyclin D/Cdk4 complex, thereby preventing the phosphorylation of RB and, in turn, halting cell cycle progression by preventing the activation of E2F. In short, p53 is a tumor suppressor gene that arrests the cell cycle when there is DNA damage. The E6 and E7 proteins work by inhibiting tumor suppression genes involved in that pathway: E6 inhibits p53, while E7 inhibits p53, p21, and RB.

E6 - This protein has a close relationship with a cellular protein called E6-AP (E6-Associated Protein). E6-AP is involved in the ubiquitin ligase pathway; a system which acts to degrade proteins. E6-AP binds ubiquitin to the p53 protein, thereby flagging it for proteosomal degradation.

Genome organization of human papillomavirus type 16, one of the subtypes known to cause cervical cancer. (E1-E7 early genes, L1-L2 late genes: capsid)

An infection with one or more high-risk HPV types is believed to be a prerequisite for the development of cervical cancer (the vast majority of HPV infections are not high risk); according to the American Cancer Society, women with no history of the virus do not develop this type of cancer. However, most HPV infections are cleared rapidly by the immune system and do not progress to cervical cancer. Because the process of transforming normal cervical cells into cancerous ones is slow, cancer occurs in people who have been infected with HPV for a long time, usually over a decade or more.[22][23]

Sexually transmitted HPVs also cause a major fraction of anal cancers and approximately 25% of cancers of the mouth and upper throat (known as the oropharynx) (see figure).[20] The latter commonly present in the tonsil area and HPV is linked to the increase in oral cancers in non-smokers.[24][25] Engaging in anal sex or oral sex with an HPV-infected partner may increase the risk of developing these types of cancers.[21]

Studies show a link between HPV infection and penile and anal cancer,[20] and the risk for anal cancer is 17 to 31 times higher among gay and bisexual men than among heterosexual men.[26][27] It has been suggested that anal Pap smear screening for anal cancer might benefit some sub-populations of men or women who engage in anal sex.[28] There is no consensus that such screening is beneficial, or who should get an anal Pap smear.[29][30]

**HEALTH**SCOUTER

# WARTS

## Skin Warts

Some HPV infections can cause warts (verrucae), which are noncancerous skin growths. Infection with these types of HPV causes a rapid growth of cells on the outer layer of the skin.[31] Types of warts include:

- Common warts: Some "cutaneous" HPV types, such as HPV-1 and HPV-2, cause *common* skin warts. Common warts are often found on the hands and feet, but can also occur in other areas, such as the elbows or knees. Common warts have a characteristic cauliflower-like surface and are typically slightly raised above the surrounding skin. Cutaneous HPV types do not usually cause genital warts and are not associated with the development of cancer.

- Plantar warts are found on the soles of the feet. Plantar warts grow inward, generally causing pain when walking.

- Subungual or periungual warts form under the fingernail (subungual), around the fingernail or on the cuticle (periungual). They may be more difficult to treat than warts in other locations.[32]

- Flat warts: Flat warts are most commonly found on the arms, face or forehead. Like common warts, flat warts occur most frequently in children and teens. In people with normal immune function, flat warts are not associated with the development of cancer.[33]

Genital warts are quite contagious, while common, flat, and plantar warts are much less likely to spread from person to person.

## Genital Warts

Genital or anal warts (condylomata acuminata or venereal warts) are the most easily recognized sign of genital HPV infection. Although a wide variety of HPV types can cause genital warts, types 6 and 11 account for about 90% of all cases.[34][35]

Most people who acquire genital wart-associated HPV types clear the infection rapidly without ever developing warts or any other symptoms. People may transmit the virus to others even if they don't display overt symptoms of infection.

HPV types that tend to cause genital warts are not the same ones that cause cervical cancer.[36] However, since an individual can be infected with multiple types of HPV, the presence of warts does not rule

# HPV: THE HUMAN PAPILLOMAVIRUS

out the possibility of high risk types of the virus also being present.

The types of HPV that cause genital warts are usually different from the types that cause warts on other parts of the body, such as the hands or inner thighs. People do not get genital warts by touching warts on their hands or feet.[37]

*I am with a person that is positive with genital warts. She hasn't had an outbreak in eight years, how am I sure I won't get it?*

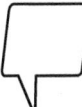
*Are you sure its genital warts or herpes? Genital warts are caused by HPV.*

*I was treated for genital warts last year and have not had any symptoms since December. I have also been fully vaccinated with the Gardasil shots. My boyfriend recently got treated for genital warts, and we are pretty sure he got it from me, as we started dating last year while I was still undergoing treatment.*

*My concern is that even though we now share the same HPV strain, will I start developing symptoms of genital warts again since he has it now? I am symptom free so far but worry that the viral shedding of the HPV cells from him will* re-infect me in a new area on my vagina or other places where I did not have genital warts treated before.

I have read that it is not possible to re-infect oneself with the same HPV strain if you already have it, but can that same HPV strain infect you in areas where you did not have genital warts before? In other words, because he now has warts, will I get new genital warts in areas where I was not exposed to and did not have symptoms before? Or has my body built up enough immunity to that strain because I have been treated for it, and because I already received the 3 Gardasil shots?

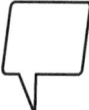From what I understand it is possible for the virus to reactivate later. It is possible for another strain of HPV to cause the same problems.

Then again, I've read (mostly here, I think I read it somewhere else) that wearing condoms can help give your body some time to heal from the HPV. The virus doesn't go away, as you know, but the viral load is reduced.

As far as can HPV affect other areas other than the original site: Absolutely.

# HPV: THE HUMAN PAPILLOMAVIRUS

 *Does having HPV mean you will get warts or cancer?*

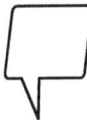 Not necessarily.

You can only get genital warts from low risk HPV. High risk HPV does not lead to genital warts.

High risk HPV can lead to cancer if:
1) The body doesn't fight the virus
2) Atypical cells are undetected
3) Atypical cells are untreated

High risk HPV doesn't guarantee cancer. Cancer from HPV is actually quite uncommon.

 *Can you pass it on to a male if genital warts go away?*

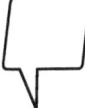 Are you asking about low risk or high risk HPV?

Either way, HPV is a virus and it stays in your body even if it isn't causing any problems. Think of it as being similar to chicken pox. The virus lives in the body, but it doesn't cause problems. If it becomes a problem later in life, then that is called Shingles.

Back to HPV. It can remain active in a person's body and he/she never knows. It is passed by *skin to skin contact, not body fluids. So, it can be passed even if the person doesn't know he/she has it. Matter of fact, that is how (I think) most HPV is spread - the person doesn't know he/she has it.*

## RESPIRATORY PAPILLOMATOSIS

HPV types 6 and 11 can cause a rare condition known as recurrent respiratory papillomatosis, in which warts form on the larynx[38] or other areas of the respiratory tract.[39][23]

These warts can recur frequently, may require repetitive surgery, may interfere with breathing, and in extremely rare cases can progress to cancer.[40][23]

**HEALTH**SCOUTER

## HPV IN IMMUNOCOMPROMISED PATIENTS

In very rare cases, HPV may cause epidermodysplasia verruciformis in immunocompromised individuals. The virus, unchecked by the immune system, causes the overproduction of keratin by skin cells, resulting in lesions resembling warts or cutaneous horns.[41]

For instance, Dede Koswara, an Indonesian man developed warts that spread across his body and became root-like growths. Attempted treatment by both Indonesian and American doctors included surgical removal of the warts.

**HEALTH**SCOUTER

## CERVICAL CANCER PREVENTION

Avoiding sexual contact with an infected person is the only 100% effective prevention method; however, many people are unaware that they are infected with HPV. Condoms offer some protection, but exposed skin can transmit the virus. Two vaccines are currently available (see "HPV vaccines" below) to women between the ages of 9 and 26.

### Pap Smear Screening

Certain types of sexually transmitted HPVs can cause cervical cancer. Persistent infection with one or more of about a dozen of these "high-risk" HPV types is an important factor in nearly all cases of cervical cancer. The development of HPV-induced cervical cancer is a slow process that generally takes many years. During this development phase, pre-cancerous cells can be detected by regular cervical cytology Papanicolaou screening, colloquially known as "Pap" smear testing. The Pap test is an effective strategy for reducing the risk of invasive cervical cancer. The Pap test involves taking cells from the cervix and putting them on a small glass slide and examining them under a microscope to look for abnormal cells. This method is 70% to 80% effective in detecting HPV-caused cellular abnormalities. A more sensitive method is a "Thin

Prep," in which the cells from the cervix are placed in a liquid solution. This test is 85% to 95% effective in detecting HPV-caused cellular abnormalities. The latter method is mainly used on women over 30. It is a combination Pap-HPV DNA test. If this test comes back negative women can usually wait 3 years before having the test done again. Detailed inspection of the cervix by colposcopy may be indicated if abnormal cells are detected by routine Pap smear. A frequently occurring example of an abnormal cell found in association with HPV is the koilocyte. (See figure.) The American College of Obstetricians and Gynecologists states that the newer liquid based cytology methods (Thinprep and Surepath) may miss 15–35% of CIN3's and cancer.

The Center for Disease Control (CDC) recommends that women get a Pap test no later than 3 years after their first sexual encounter and no later than 21 years of age. Women should have a Pap test every year until age 30. After age 30, women should discuss risk factors with their health care provider to determine whether a Pap test should be done yearly. If risk factors are low and previous Pap tests have been negative, most women only need to have tests every 2–3 years until 65 years of age (Centers for Disease Control 2005). All women are encouraged to get a yearly Pap smear solely to detect cellular abnormalities caused by HPV.[42]

Since the Pap test was developed there has been a 70% decrease in cervical cancer deaths over the last 50 years. Pap smear testing has proven to be one of the most successful screening tests in the history of medicine.

A study published in April 2007 suggests that the act of performing a Pap smear produces an inflammatory cytokine response, which may initiate immunologic clearance of HPV, therefore reducing the risk of cervical cancer. Women who had even a single Pap smear in their history had a lower incidence of cancer. "A statistically significant decline in the HPV positivity rate correlated with the lifetime number of Pap smears received."[43]

*I just had a Pap smear and my first abnormal result. My doctor wants me to test again in six months but said that I don't have HPV which she said is really good. I also have to get a pelvic ultrasound done now because she felt some fullness on the one side and wanted to make sure. She said the two issues are not related but I'm really worried, what could this be caused by? I just am getting over a flu virus and I my period*

just ended when I got the exam and she said that could cause it (just coming off a period). I hope I don't have cancer!

> If you had even a chance of cancer my dear they would have sent you for more tests to determine that fact rather than telling you to wait six months. If you feel in your heart that there may be that chance, then I urge you to ask to be either re tested by the same doctor or seek a second opinion for some peace of mind!.

> Please do yourself a big, big favor and DO NOT read anything regarding cervical cancer that you do not need to. Some good reading for you would be to Google the word "cervical dysplasia", and its suitable treatment etc. That might bring some knowledge for you that will explain what is going on with your abnormal Pap smears.

I have been with my husband for 23 years. Three years ago I had a normal Pap smear with no HPV detected. This month I had an abnormal Pap smear with HPV detected. Could this virus have been dormant in my body for more than 23 years?

# HPV: THE HUMAN PAPILLOMAVIRUS

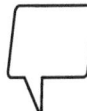
*Yes it can remain dormant for decades. After I had my first invasive cancer in 1991, it was dormant for 15 years before returning again in 2006. What type of HPV do you have, high risk or low risk and what types? If you don't know this info, ask your doctor's office and get copies of your test results (you should always do this). Depending on your answers will determine the course of treatment going forward.*

*My Pap smear was ASCUS. I had a second pap and HPV done yesterday. All my other Pap smears were normal. I know they have only been testing Pap smears with HPV for the last five or so years. So it is possible to actually have the virus but shows up negative?*

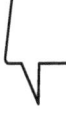
*Not all doctors automatically have the HPV test done with the Pap smear. Many only have the HPV test run if the Pap smear is positive, others have it done regardless. Since HPV affects basically the entire genital system and not just the cervix you can have a negative Pap smear, yet have HPV elsewhere, say the vagina which can at a later point spread to the cervix. When you get your results, make sure to find out exactly what strains of HPV you have.*

*Is it normal to have vaginal warts?*

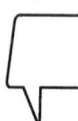
*Not if they're truly warts. There's a STD called HPV human papillomavirus. It needs to be treated by a doctor.*

*If that's what you have, they need to be removed by a gynecologist. I had them and was diagnosed with HPV years ago, only found out through a Pap smear. Must be treated and then you would have a Pap smear every year to check for abnormalities.*

*I'm really terrified of this result. I had a nurse talk to me in person about it and she said that if had just been an ASCUS result and no HPV that she wouldn't worry about it, but since I tested for high risk HPV that she wants to schedule a colposcopy. Aside from worrying about the pain of a biopsy and endocervical cutterage, (read horror stories) I'm deathly afraid of the outcome.*

*She said (and I quote) that an ASCUS result is actually a good thing. She said that it is 1 step away from 'normal' results and that even though the Pap smear is just a screening tool, if there were cancer cells that they would have probably been able to spot them. She also said that she has never seen an ASCUS result from a Pap smear come back as worse than low-grade-- that it is rare for an atypical result to actually be cancer (because the cells look almost normal) She ALSO said that when she did my pap, I didn't bleed and that my cervix looked healthy (and that she has seen ones that she could tell weren't good)*

*Can someone ease my mind and/or be honest with me? Is she just trying to make me less scared?*

*Before this, (and I'm 26 years old) I had NEVER had a pap, been sexually active for six years- --what if I have cancer??!! What if it has been brewing this whole time since I became sexually active???? I mean, I have seen posts all over the place that said different things. One lady scared the crap out of me by saying that HER doctor told her that high risk HPV with ASCUS result means 80% cancer chance!!!!!!!*

*My mom said it is rare for someone my age to have cervical cancer and that it takes about 10 years to become cancer in HPV patients... but my defense is that Jade Goody died at age 27 from cervical cancer.*

*Help me please... I'm making myself sick with worry. I am so scared about what the biopsy will say. Can a pap really tell if there is cancer? If so, why the colposcopy? I understand it is to monitor...and I'm going to go get it done in about two weeks... but OMG what if it IS cancer?*

I understand your fears and worries, but I think at this point your doctor just needs more information. The best way to do that is with the colposcopy. The doctor will probably take a biopsy of the exocervix. The doctor might, if he/she has reason to, do an ECC.

There are several steps between your pap results and cancer, for most women. There are rare cases. My suggestion, as a woman who was diagnosed with cervical cancer last year... is take it one step at a time. Worrying only gives your mind something to do - and it isn't productive.

My suggestions are to read reputable sites (CDC, etc), learn the basics of what will happen. Try to avoid horror stories. Write down your questions and leave room for writing answers.

My honest opinion is that no one knows until the colposcopy and biopsy reports are back.

*I can't (and won't) make predictions, if for no other reason than I was on the wrong end of a prediction!*

*From what I've read, I would say that statistics and percentages are on the side of the ASCUS being the beginning stages of atypical cells. Caught early, atypical cells of the cervix are very easily treated. Sometimes they are left to let the body heal itself (especially if the woman is younger than 30). If the body doesn't heal itself, then the colposcopy and biopsy often remove all atypical cells. If that doesn't take care of it, then sometimes a cone type biopsy (LEEP or CKC) is done. Often, that removes all atypical cells. If not, then further investigation is done.*

*Most cervical cancer (80%) is squamous cell. Squamous cell carcinoma is very easily (because of biology) found (by the pap or colposcopy) and it is usually very easily treated (by biopsy or cone). IF found early and treated/biopsied.*

*It is possible that the ASCUS is from an infection of some sort. That is why the ASCUS= undetermined significance.*

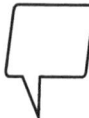 *First off, wherever you read that an HPV+ and ASCUS pap has an 80% chance of being cancer is just plain wrong.*

*I first had an HPV+ and ASCUS Pap smear about two years ago (wow! time flies!). I also had missed my Pap smears for over five years at that point (I'm 32 now) so I know EXACTLY where you are coming from right now. I was terrified that I had already developed cancer since it had been so long since I had a pap.*

*In my countless hours of internet search on this topic, I have been able to pull some statistics together that put my mind somewhat at ease through all of this:*

*I guess what I found comforting about this was to look at how many thousands of women each year are treated for high-grade cervical cell changes versus how many are actually diagnosed with invasive cancer - it's a pretty low percent. So, even if your colposcopy diagnoses CIN II or III, the chances that it can be treated prior to actual cancer developing is really quite good!*

*Now, as for me, like I had mentioned, two years ago I had the HPV+ and ASCUS pap. Since I was going to my normal general practitioner and not an actual gynecologist, I don't think she was totally up to speed on the appropriate follow up care for such a result because normally a doctor would recommend a colposcopy (like yours has), but she kept giving me Pap smears every four months for almost a year before she recommended I see an actual gynecologist for a colposcopy. I did that last May and the results came back as CIN I and the gynecologist prescribed the "wait and see approach" as CIN I has a good chance (as noted above) of regressing without treatment.*

*Well, my next pap in November of this year once again came back HPV+ and ASC-H, which is basically an ASCUS pap but with a suspicion of high-grade changes. I had the colposcopy done once again, this time the biopsy came back as CIN III. So, I had a LEEP done earlier this month where the doctor removed FOUR areas of CIN III but found, thank god, no actual cancer.*

*So, I guess my lessons that I took away from this are:*

*1. I will never, ever miss another pap in my life.*
*2. Educate yourself on this topic as much as possible. There is a lot of misinformation out*

there and unfortunately even doctors don't seem to be entirely up to speed on this issue, but if you stick with reputable sites, such as the American Journal of Obstetrics and Gynecology, you will get some really good info.

3. You have to be your own advocate. I scheduled multiple consultations with my doctor JUST to ask questions. If you don't understand something, ask. Don't worry about being a pest. It is your body and your right to know as much as possible about what is going on and why certain recommendations are being made. No one else is going to do this for you.

4. If you are not comfortable with your current doctor, find a new one. Cervical cancer issues are usually very slow moving. This doesn't mean that you can ignore any problems, but does allow for some time to get a doctor you are comfortable with.

I know that the Jane Goody story is scary - she died just prior to my last colposcopy and I was absolutely terrified that I was going to be in the same boat - but the average statistical age for cervical cancer is the mid 40's and 50's, so if you are catching any precursors now, you are most likely in really good shape!

# HPV: THE HUMAN PAPILLOMAVIRUS

*Last Tuesday, I got back my Pap smear results and was diagnosed with HPV. I'm having a really, really hard time dealing with it. My gynecologist just wanted to say "It's really common" over and over again and instead of making me feel better about it, it just made my anxiety and worry even stronger every time she said it.*

*I understand it is very common, and I am coming here in hopes someone who's been diagnosed as well can give me some advice as to how to cope with learning you have HPV.*

*I'm 21 and I've only had sex with two people in my life. My ex (of four years) and my fiancé.*

*My fiancé and I have already had sex (and so I know it's possible he could be the one who gave it to me...or I could have gave it to him) so he has it as well. He's been very sympathetic and still wants to marry me and still says he loves me no matter what but I'm having such a hard time dealing with having it. I just feel dirty.*

*My fiancé always tells me I'm not; I'm still the same person. But I just don't feel it. I felt so alive before I found out I have HPV. And I have so* many questions about HPV because I've talked to my gynecologist and looked on Web sites but there's still so many things I don't understand.

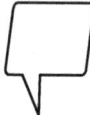

The main thing though even after all the questions is just I really don't understand how to deal with it. It's on my mind every day, every minute, every second, after I wake up.

Your immune system can control this virus. Make sure you take a good multivitamin, eat lots of antioxidant foods. Example-- broccoli, blueberries, tomatoes, red grapes, garlic, spinach, carrots --- vitamins A, C, E, folic acid. Stop smoking.

HPV can be treated when caught early. It's not the end of the world. You are so young. You are getting the shot. You have a fiancé. You will be fine.

Someone told me once--- Think of it as a really bad cold--- HPV is a virus that is treatable. Imagine if we didn't know? At least doctors are now able to test, treat and sometimes cure it. Or sometimes your immune system fights it off after a couple of years.

Do abnormal cells in a Pap smear test mean HPV positive?

# HPV: THE HUMAN PAPILLOMAVIRUS

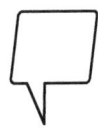 *An abnormal pap could be several things besides HPV. It could be an infection of some sort, recent trauma (like from intercourse), various products used near/in the vagina like lubrication, etc. OR it could be from HPV.*

**HEALTH**SCOUTER

## HPV TESTING

The HPV test detects many common "low" and "high-risk" HPV genotypes. This test is an important screening option, since a doctor may recommend more frequent Pap testing if the HPV test is positive for "high-risk" HPV. In March 2003, the US FDA approved a "hybrid-capture" test, marketed by Digene, as a primary screening tool for detecting HPV. This test was also approved for use as an adjunct to Pap testing, and may be performed during a routine Pap smear.

When patients are screened with both HPV testing and Pap testing the sensitivity reaches 100%. HPV testing can diagnose CIN 2-3 among women older than 30 years.[44] The sensitivity of HPV testing alone was 94.6% and specificity was 94.1%. For patients at similar risk to those in this study (0.4% had CIN 2-3), this leads to a positive predictive value of 6.0% and negative predictive value of 100.0% (click here to adjust these results for patients at higher or lower risk of CIN 2-3).

The CDC states on its "STD Facts-HPV Vaccine" page that "An HPV test or a Pap test can tell that a woman may have HPV, but these tests cannot tell the specific HPV type(s) that a woman has."[42]

In Australia, a self-sampling HPV DNA test - that women can do at home using an ordinary tampon - is being marketed by Tam Pap. It has been approved by the Therapeutic Goods Administration for distribution in Australia.

The recent outcomes in the identification of molecular pathways involved in cervical cancer provide helpful information about novel biomarkers that allow monitoring these essential molecular events in histological or cytological specimens. These biomarkers are likely to improve the detection of lesions that have a high risk of progression in both primary screening and triage settings. E6 and E7 mRNA detection (HPV OncoTect) or p16 cell-cycle protein levels are examples of these new molecular markers. According to published results these markers, which are highly sensitive and specific, allow to identify cells going through malignant transformation.[45]

 *I tested positive for HPV last year, then tested negative 6 months later. This year I tested positive again. Does that mean it's still in my body, or that I got it again?*

# HPV: THE HUMAN PAPILLOMAVIRUS

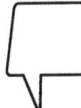
*Once you have been exposed to HPV the virus remains in your body. The HPV test (and I assume you mean the DNA test) detects active infections.*

*It is possible that your second positive test is from the same virus being detected again (therefore your body didn't completely fight it) OR (and this is more likely) you have another strain of HPV causing problems.*

*I've been married 24 years and neither of us have ever had an extramarital affair... last two years Pap smear nothing detected.*

*My 2009 Pap smear detected HPV... where did this come from?*

*I understand your worry and concern.*

*I assume either you or your husband had had some sort of sexual experience prior to getting together (24 years ago). I assume this because HPV is spread by skin to skin contact; in this case, genital skin to genital skin contact. Some people are fortunate and can make it so the virus doesn't cause problems. Others aren't so lucky. High risk HPV can stay in the body, and be active for months, years, or even decades.*

*I also suspect this pap is the first time your doctor did the HPV test during your Pap smears.*

*I was in a very similar situation. January 2008 I got the results from my pap. My pap smear test was fine, just has it has been for the past 24 years. The HPV test, which my doctor did for the very first time, came back positive for high risk HPV. There is a bit of a long story, and I am a very rare case, but I don't go into the details. Suffice it to say that I am VERY glad my doctor did the HPV test.*

## HPV TESTING IN MALES

Although it is possible to test for HPV DNA in men,[46] there are no FDA-approved tests for general screening in the United States[26] or tests approved by the Canadian government[47], since the testing is inconclusive and considered medically unnecessary.[48]

Genital warts are the only visible sign of low-risk HPV in men, and can be identified with a visual check of the genital area. These visible growths, however, are the result of non-carcinogenic HPV types. 5% acetic acid (vinegar) is used to identify both warts and squamous intraepithelial neoplasia (SIL) lesions with limited success[26] by causing abnormal tissue to appear white, but most doctors have found this technique helpful only in moist areas, such as the female genital tract.[26]

*I am currently 34 years old. I have over the course of my life had sex with over 400 women. In all but about 10 cases it was ALWAYS protected no matter what happened. I am very aware of avoiding STIs and even though have been very tempted not to wear a condom at points, I have ALWAYS used condoms for both oral, vaginal anal sex etc. I am a little unclear*

about "skin to skin" contact (does that mean fluid to skin also (?) or simply brushing up against someone intimately) that is referred too since wearing a condom is not 100% protection as there is the scrotum and labia that can and do touch even when wearing a condom.

So I can assume that having slept with so many women that I have contracted some forms of HPV.

I have no symptoms other than itchy skin, but this could be simply dryness. I've had verrucas on my feet and "hard patches" of skin on my hands. Now I am getting worried about HPV since the incubation period seems to be such a long time and there is no "cure" for the strains. I have now since married, had kids, and cannot possibly imagine what risk I am putting my wife under. I re-iterate I have no genital warts, nor ever had any. I would like some advice about what course of action to take. I see some clinics offering HPV testing for men, yet most sites state that testing for men doesn't make sense.

I do however need to know that since I've always worn a condom and IF I did have some strains of HPV on (for example) my scrotum, and myself and my wife had unprotected sex, does that put

# HPV: THE HUMAN PAPILLOMAVIRUS

*her at the immediate risk of contracting the high risk HPV that leads to cervical cancer or would the HPV stay outside her body. You can imagine the last thing I want to be responsible for...*

*So, A) can men have any tests that are reliable and B) with my history of partners protected sex and no symptoms what would be the best course of action for me and my wife. C) Can I get tested?*

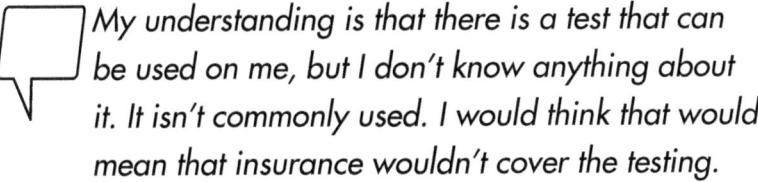

My understanding is that there is a test that can be used on me, but I don't know anything about it. It isn't commonly used. I would think that would mean that insurance wouldn't cover the testing.

HPV lives in the skin, not in the blood or other fluids. It can be transmitted, like you suggested, from scrotum to labia or anus even if condoms are used (just as one example).

I don't know what advice to give you. All I can say is that your wife has essentially slept with everyone you have slept with because whatever (if anything) you got from them you could potentially pass along to her.

I would suggest she let her doctor know of her exposure (via you). If I were her I'd be asking for an HPV test at my next pap. If, for any reasons she needs a colposcopy she needs to request an ECC (endocervical curettage). She needs to stay current on her Pap smears, religiously.

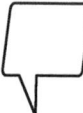
I am a gay male with HPV. There is a test that can determine whether you have HPV, so I have read. I think it is a blood test. My understanding of HPV is that it is in your DNA, or something like that, so that's why it is so hard to 'cure'. So I have read something where they said there are two tests. One will tell you if you have HPV, the other will tell you what strain of HPV you have. You really need to find out, as if it is high risk you need to act on it now to prevent it from progressing to cancer, or keep an eye on it so that when it does turn to cancer you know early. And I would suggest that your wife goes for a Pap smear ASAP. Knowing as much as possible about this is a must and will help.

## HPV VACCINES

On June 8, 2006, the US Food and Drug Administration approved Gardasil, a prophylactic HPV vaccine which is marketed by Merck. The vaccine trial,[49] conducted in adult women with a mean age of 23, showed protection against initial infection with HPV types 16 and 18, which together cause 70% of cervical cancers, and can cause other cancers, such as anal cancer. The vaccine also protects against HPV types 6 and 11, which cause 90 percent of genital warts.

GlaxoSmithKline is seeking approval for a prophylactic vaccine known as Cervarix targeting HPV types 16 and 18. It is delivered in three shots over six months. It is intended for females from 10 years of age onwards.[50]

Gardasil vaccine is delivered in a series of three shots over six months at a cost of approximately $360 (US dollars). The CDC recommends that girls and women between the ages of 11 and 26 be vaccinated,[42] though girls as young as 9 may benefit.[51] Females not yet sexually active can be expected to receive the full benefit of vaccination. Women over 26 can be vaccinated at the discretion of a doctor, but the vaccination has not yet been approved by the FDA for this age range, and may not be covered by insurance.

Studies have not yet conclusively shown benefits for patients over 26, possibly due to the high prevalence of infection and the fact that the vaccine has no effect upon current infections.

HPV vaccine is made up of proteins from the outer coat of the virus (HPV). There is no infectious material in this vaccine. There is also no thimerosal, a mercury based preservative, in the HPV vaccine.[42] This vaccine has been tested in over 11,000 females (ages 9–26 years) around the world. These studies have shown no serious side effects. The most common side effect is soreness at the injection site. CDC, working with the FDA, will continue to monitor the safety of the vaccine after it is in general use.[52]

The vaccine does not appear to protect against HPV types that females are infected with at the time of vaccination. However, females already infected with one or more vaccine HPV types before vaccination would be protected against disease caused by the other vaccine HPV types covered by the vaccine. Therefore, although overall vaccine effectiveness would be lower when administered to females who have been sexually active, and would decrease with age and likelihood of HPV exposure with increasing number of sex partners, the majority of females in this age group will derive at least partial benefit from vaccination. The vaccine will not have any therapeutic effect on existing HPV infection or cervical lesions.[53]

Since the current vaccine will not protect women against all the HPV types that cause cervical cancer, women should continue to seek Pap smear testing, even after receiving the vaccine. Cervical cancer screening recommendations have not changed for females who receive HPV vaccine.[53]

Both men and women are carriers of HPV.[54] Possible benefits and efficacy of vaccinating men are being studied.

In addition to preventive vaccines, laboratory research and several human clinical trials are focused on the development of therapeutic HPV vaccines. In general, these vaccines focus on the main HPV oncogenes E6 and E7. Since expression of E6 and E7 is required for promoting the growth of cervical cancer cells (and cells within warts), it is hoped that immune responses against the two oncogenes might eradicate established tumors.[55]

 *Wow, I was reading about the possibility that Gardasil increases the chance of CIN2/3 in women who are HPV positive, and I was*

*FREAKED OUT! I just received my last dose of the vaccine yesterday!!!!!*

*I found the study, read it, and it actually made me feel much better. So here's my executive summary:*

*First, the link to FDA (government NOT commercial) website with the study results:*

*http://www.fda.gov/ohrms/dockets/ac/06/briefing/2006-4222B3.pdf*

*Start on page 13: "Concerns Regarding Primary Endpoint Analyses among Subgroups".*

*Okay, so some of the women in the studies were "seropostive" aka they had HPV antibodies in their blood and some were "PCR positive" aka a positive HPV DNA test. And some were positive for both.*

*For women who were both PCR positive and seropostive in study 013: the placebo group 7.7% developed CIN 2/3 compared with 11.1% in the Gardasil group. That's a bit concerning!*

*But then they talk about how this group of women was a "subgroup" of the study and so they hadn't made it demographically even. For example, 6.5% of the Gardasil group had previously had an HGSIL result from a pap, while only 3.7% in the placebo group did. And in the Gardasil group there were more smokers and more women with other STDs.*

*In study 015, the women in the PCR/seropostive subgroup were more demographically even, and the placebo group had a CIN 2/3 rate of 6.3% and in the Gardasil group it was 6.0%.*

*So basically they conclude that this issue warrants "more study" but it appears that study 013 was probably just messed up demographically.*

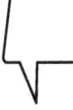
Just goes to show that everything must be taken in "context". So often people just jump to conclusions and don't read or don't understand the data. Then they run around talking about how you can get cancer from the vaccine. Fact is there is absolutely no HPV DNA in the vaccine at all. Unlike some vaccines which are produced by attenuating (weakening) the organism, this is not the case with Gardasil. It is made from VLP's, virus like particles so it cannot convey the HPV DNA to anyone only work to stimulate an antibody response.

*I really think that there is a huge issue with credibility. If you read someone's blog and take it as law, that only perpetuates fear and conspiracy. If you take the time to do the research, learn about the issue and then create a stance, I think the argument becomes mature and credible. Particularly regarding health, we need to be cautious about the potential panic we're imposing upon someone who is just beginning to learn about these issues. I think it is irresponsible to haphazardly post without validating that the information is accurate.*

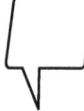

*You know, when I searched online to try and find answers, I came across several papers basically saying that Gardasil increased your risk of CIN 2/3 if you already had HPV. There is a particularly bad one from "Judicial Watch." (After reading more stuff from their site, I have come to the conclusion that they think everything is government conspiracy.) Their report is full of these anecdotal stories of girls developing huge outbreaks of warts and others suddenly dying after getting the vaccine.*

*But when it talks about the increase of in CIN 2/3 cases, it cites back to that FDA document I was talking about. It also doesn't mention that the* "adverse reaction" events were about the same as in the placebo group for everything except injection site reaction.

> Totally get the vaccine. With the exception of the one group discussed in that study, everything I've seen seems to show positive results for the vaccine in HPV positive women. This applies to both clearance rates and the rates of developing dysplasia.

Usually the differences are very small, even fractions of percentage points. The studies usually conclude that there is no difference. However, it seems to me that since the vaccinated group pretty much always comes out slightly ahead, the vaccine would be a good thing!

# HEALTHSCOUTER

# HPV: THE HUMAN PAPILLOMAVIRUS

## CONDOMS

The Centers for Disease Control and Prevention says that "While the effect of condoms in preventing HPV infection is unknown, condom use has been associated with a lower rate of cervical cancer, an HPV-associated disease."[36]

According to Marcus Steiner and Willard Cates in the New England Journal of Medicine, "the protection that condoms offer cannot be precisely quantified."[56] However, in a study reported in the same issue,[57] of 82 female university students followed for eight months, the incidence of genital HPV infection was 37.8 per 100 patient-years among women whose partners used condoms for all instances of intercourse, compared with 89.3 per 100 patient-years in women whose partners used condoms less than 5% of the time. The researchers concluded that "Among newly sexually active women, consistent condom use by their partners appears to reduce the risk of cervical and vulvovaginal HPV infection."

Other studies have suggested that regular condom use can effectively limit the ongoing persistence and spread of HPV to additional genital sites in individuals who are already infected.[58][59]

Thus, condom use may reduce the risk that infected individuals will progress to cervical cancer or develop additional genital warts. Planned Parenthood recommends condom use to reduce the risk of contracting HPV.[60]

*Can I get HPV if I use a condom?*

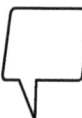
*Yes. HPV is spread by skin to skin contact, not body fluids. A condom does not cover all skin which can have contact during sexual acts.*

## MICROBICIDES

Ongoing research has suggested that several inexpensive chemicals might serve to block HPV transmission if applied to the genitals prior to sexual contact.[61] These candidate agents, known as topical microbicides, are currently undergoing clinical efficacy testing. A recent study indicates that some sexual lubricant brands that use a gelling agent called carrageenan can inhibit papillomavirus infection in vitro.[62]

Clinical trials are needed to determine whether carrageenan-based sexual lubricant gels are effective for blocking the sexual transmission of HPVs in vivo.

## TREATMENT

There is currently no cure or treatment for HPV infection.[63][42]

*Therapies for conditions caused by HPV are addressed in main chapter covering the various HPV-related diseases.*

**HEALTH**SCOUTER

# HPV VACCINE

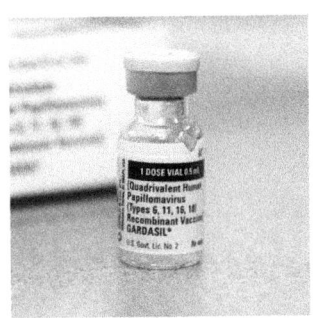

Human papillomavirus (HPV) vaccine is a vaccine that prevents infection with certain species of human papillomavirus associated with the development of cervical cancer, genital warts,[1] and some less common cancers (e.g., anal,[2] vulvar,[3] vaginal,[3] penile[2]). Two HPV vaccines are currently on the market: Gardasil and Cervarix.[4] Both vaccines protect against two of the HPV types that cause cervical cancer, and some other genital cancers; Gardasil also protects against two of the HPV types that cause genital warts.[1]

Public health officials in Australia, Canada, Europe and United States recommend vaccination of young women against HPV to prevent cervical cancer and genital warts, and to reduce the number of painful and costly treatments for cervical dysplasia, which is caused by HPV.[5] Worldwide, HPV is the most common sexually transmitted infection in adults.[6]

For example, more than 80% of American women will have contracted at least one strain of HPV by age fifty.[7][8][9][10][11]

Although most women infected with genital HPV will not have complications from the virus,[12] worldwide there are an estimated 470,000 new cases of cervical cancer that result in 233,000 deaths per year.[13] About eighty percent of deaths from cervical cancer occur in poor countries.[14] In the United States, most of the approximately 11,000 cervical cancers found annually[15] occur in women who have never had a Pap smear, or not had one in the previous five years.

Since the vaccine only covers some high-risk types of HPV, experts still recommend regular Pap smear screening even after vaccination.[16]

Gardasil has been shown to also be effective in males, though it has not yet been approved by the FDA to be marketed as such.[2]

*If you have received an ASCUS pap, it means that abnormal cells were detected on the cervix. This can be a result of an infection as well, so it is import to follow up with your physician.*

# HPV: THE HUMAN PAPILLOMAVIRUS

*LGSIL: (Also called CIN I) mild dysplasia has been detected. Also includes cell changes caused by HPV (Human papillomavirus)*

*HGSIL: This type of result is divided into two categories:*

*Moderate Dysplasia: (also called CIN II) abnormal cells make up ½ of the thickness surface lining*

*Severe Dysplasia: (also called CIN III, or carcinoma in situ) the entire thickness of the epithelium (surface cell layer) is composed of abnormal cells but cells have not spread below the surface.*

*In my case, I had abnormal test results. I tried to call the nurses at my doctor's office but they would not answer any questions. They left a message and had the doc call me back. He told me not to worry that sometimes it goes away by itself and the next pap could be negative.*

*I had a pap and it said mild dysplasia with effects of HPV. Then I had a biopsy and it said moderate dysplasia. Now going for LEEP procedure. How serious is this and am I likely at this point to get cancer??*

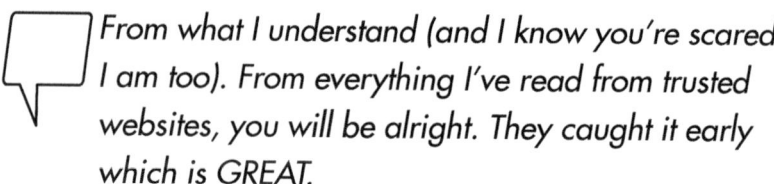
From what I understand (and I know you're scared, I am too). From everything I've read from trusted websites, you will be alright. They caught it early which is GREAT.

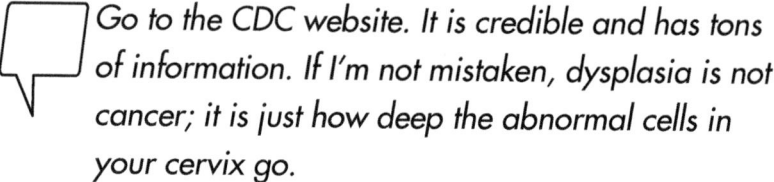
Go to the CDC website. It is credible and has tons of information. If I'm not mistaken, dysplasia is not cancer; it is just how deep the abnormal cells in your cervix go.

Cervical dysplasia is a term used to describe the appearance of abnormal cells on the surface of the cervix, the lowest part of the uterus. These changes in cervical tissue are classified as mild, moderate, or severe. While dysplasia itself does not cause health problems, it is considered to be a precancerous condition. Left untreated, dysplasia sometimes progresses to an early form of cancer known as cervical carcinoma in situ, and eventually to invasive cervical cancer.

It can take ten years or longer for cervical dysplasia to develop into cancer. Dysplasia can be detected from a Pap smear, the single most important step that a woman can take to prevent cervical cancer.

*Mild dysplasia is the most common form, and up to 70% of these cases regress on their own (i.e., the cervical tissue returns to normal without treatment). Moderate and severe dysplasia is less likely to self-resolve and have a higher rate of progression to cancer. The greater the abnormality, the higher the risk for developing cervical cancer.*

*Cervical dysplasia does not cause symptoms; therefore, regular screening and early diagnosis are important. Detecting and treating dysplasia early is essential to prevent cancer. For this reason, most physicians quickly remove suspicious cervical lesions and require frequent Pap smears to monitor for recurrences.*

## *Incidence and Prevalence*

Every year, between 250,000 and 1 million women in the United States are diagnosed with cervical dysplasia. While it can occur at any age, the peak incidence is in women between the ages of 25 to 35. Most dysplasia cases can be cured with proper treatment and follow-up. Without treatment, 30% to 50% may progress to invasive cancer.

## Risk Factors

Risk factors increase the frequency of occurrence. Several risk factors have been linked to dysplasia including multiple sexual partners, early onset of sexual activity, cigarette smoking, and sexually transmitted diseases, especially human papillomavirus (HPV) and HIV infection.

## HPV Infection

Eighty to ninety percent of women with cervical dysplasia have an HPV infection. Human papillomavirus (HPV) is a group of more than 80 different viral strains. About one-third are sexually transmitted, and some types cause genital warts. HPV infects about 25 million people in the United States, and most of the viral strains are harmless.

However, the NIH Consensus Conference on Cancer of the Cervix and the World Health Organization (WHO) have concluded that several strains of HPV cause cervical cancer. The strains found most frequently in precancerous lesions and in cervical cancer are types 16 and 18. Other strains with high malignant potential include 31, 33, 35, 39, 45, 51, 52, 56, 58, and 68, and together, they account for almost 90% of cancerous lesions and dysplasia in HPV infections.

# HPV: THE HUMAN PAPILLOMAVIRUS

Most HPV infections resolve within six months and many women develop immunity. HPV often does not cause symptoms. One study found that nearly one-half of the women infected with HPV had no symptoms and a person may not even know that they are infected. Untreated HPV can result in recurrent and persistent cervical dysplasia and many experts believe that HPV is the main cause for changes in cervical cells that result in dysplasia.

*I was just diagnosed this week with severe cervical dysplasia and I have tested negative for HPV twice (actually 3 times including once several years ago). I had never had an abnormal pap in my life until late last year. My doctor, as soon as I had the abnormal pap, recommended a re-pap within a month (I ended up waiting until January to go in though). That pap too came back abnormal, so they did a procedure called a colposcopy where they look at your cervix and possibly take a sample for biopsy. When they did the biopsy they thought I had maybe mild dysplasia... but then I got the call saying it is CIN III, the most severe form without being actual invasive cancer. And again, I don't have HPV, so it's very unusual.*

 I have to go in for a pelvic ultrasound next week because she felt fullness on the one side and wanted to make sure it was ok so maybe I would know more after that? She said the two weren't related.

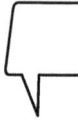 The swelling could be from many different things: endometriosis, andyomyosis, cysts, bowel problems, etc. The ultrasound will help determine a possible cause.

The rechecking with the pap in 4–6 months is fairly standard if the doctor suspects mild dysplasia. Is your doctor running a separate HPV/NDA test? I believe the most commonly used one is by Digene (company name).

It is possible to have cervical dysplasia and not have HPV, though it is usually found, later, that there is/was HPV infection.

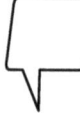 I suggest that if/when your doctor performs a colposcopy for you to request an ECC (endocervical curettage) at that time. It checks the cells that are further up in the cervix which cannot be sampled during a pap or colposcopy.

 How reliable are the statistics that mild dysplasia will turn to severe dysplasia then cancer?

# HPV: THE HUMAN PAPILLOMAVIRUS

> I don't know what the chances are of moderate dysplasia developing into cancer but I do know that about 70% of cases of mild dysplasia resolve on their own within two years. I've had mild dysplasia now for three years and it has yet to progress.

> Just want to share my story - I was diagnosed with CIN I almost exactly a year ago. However, I changed doctors a few months later and when my 6-month follow-up Pap smear came back abnormal again, the new doctor insisted on doing another colposcopy to "see for herself". Well, I'm glad she did, because she found four areas that came back as CIN III!!!! She would not say outright whether the CIN had progressed from CIN I to CIN III in a matter of months OR that the previous doctor had missed the more significant areas of dysplasia during my first colposcopy.
>
> I truly believe that it was the latter case due to two reasons: my Pap smears were coming back consistently as ASC-H (before and after first biopsy) which points to the CIN III. Also, the first doctor was a total whack job.
>
> I guess my advice is to keep on top of your follow ups. Even if a significant lesion was missed during

*the colposcopy, cervical cancer usually progresses so slowly that a follow up test will catch it in time. Can I ask - what did your pap come back as? If it was ASC-H or HGSIL and your biopsy only showed CIN I, I would keep an even closer eye on it if I were you.*

*My doctor said my pap came back as A-typical abnormal cells, and the biopsy came back CIN I*

*I'm totally impressed that everyone here knows so much. My first abnormal pap was 18 years ago. I ended up with a colposcopy. I never knew there were different levels of abnormal. I don't think I had another abnormal pap until about 5 years ago- it must have been low grade, then last August I had a colposcopy, low grade, then in Feb- high grade. It didn't take long for me this time around. All this time, I had no idea that HPV was responsible, I thought all of the abnormal results were false positives. Right now, I'll go back for a pap every three months.*

*I should probably quit reading the Internet, because I read some articles where they feel like if dysplasia is found in the endocervical canal that they should do a cone.*

# HPV: THE HUMAN PAPILLOMAVIRUS

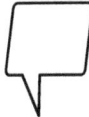 *We've discussed this a couple times in other threads, but even if the ECC comes back the positive for dysplasia, you shouldn't be too worried.*

*ECCs have a high false positive rate when you have dysplasia on the outside of your cervix because some of the dysplasia contaminates the curette as it is passing through the opening of your cervix. What the ECC is really testing for is glandular changes. If you have glandular changes, a cone would be recommended, but there's no evidence of that! The ECC is just to make sure because, like I said, your doctor can't actually see up there to see if anything is wrong.*

*I had two ASCUS Pap tests and two negative HPV tests, and then had a colposcopy done a few months later, which shows CIN 1 (mild dysplasia) with HPV changes on the ECC well as 2 spots on the outside of the cervix. My doctor has given me the choice of a LEEP/CONE but also says he is very comfortable with a wait and see approach and to repeat the Pap smear in four months. I have not yet decided what I am going to do. From what my doctor says, the HPV test will show if you have high risk HPV. Says since mine was negative for high risk the HPV changes are from a low risk* virus. I would want to know if it were high risk or not.

I have had abnormal Pap smears for the last three years. I just had a colposcopy and my results showed fragments of low grade atypical cells endocervical.

My doctor recommends another pap in six months. She didn't seem concerned.

I also asked her about an HPV test...she said "not necessary. If you have LGSIL or HGSIL, then we know you have HPV. We treat you according to results of the colposcopy, etc. So no need for the HPV test."

Are there any symptoms of HPV that I should look out for?

Are you asking about low risk or high risk HPV? I only have personal experience with high risk HPV. I had no symptoms.

If a woman has HPV can she give it to her partner just from oral sex?

Low risk HPV or high risk HPV? Either way, yes.

HPV lives in the skin, not in the body fluids.

# HPV: THE HUMAN PAPILLOMAVIRUS

*Is HPV (genital warts) a form or strain of herpes?*

No. Though they both are STDs.

*What are the pros and cons of having a LEEP? I have been diagnosed with LGSIL with HPV changes (whatever that means!). My doctor gave me the choice of wait and see or LEEP. Keep going back and forth in my mind of what to do. Opinions appreciated!*

The LEEP is an electrically charged wire that cuts away cervical tissue. The biopsy sample is cone-like (kind of) in shape). It is wider at the base (where the doctor scrapes a pap) and cuts up into the cervical canal; it biopsies the upper parts of the cervix in addition to the outer cervix.

I think the LEEP is preferred if there is squamous cell dysplasia. A Cold Knife Cone (CKC) is generally preferred by doctors if glandular cell dysplasia is suspected.

Here is my info, I am 47 years old. Here is what has been going on…

1. January 2008, uterine biopsy done for heavy bleeding results were benign hyperplasia. treatment with birth control pills. Before it was brought under control I became severely anemic.
2. July 2008, anemia resolved.
3. December 2008, uterine biopsy is normal, my doctor also did an ECC, this was also normal BUT Pap smear was ASCUS, HPV negative
4. March 2009, repeat PAP still ASCUS again negative HPV
5. April 2009, Colposcopy done,

LGSIL with HPV change (mild dysplasia)

ECC also done same results LGSIL with HPV changes (mild dysplasia)

My doctor says he is very comfortable taking a wait and see approach, BUT he will do a LEEP procedure if I want it. He says if I were a 20 year old he wouldn't suggest the LEEP but since I am no longer interested in having kids it would be OK.

Looking for opinions as to others experiences or what they would do if given the same results.

# HPV: THE HUMAN PAPILLOMAVIRUS

*Wondering about the contradictions where the ECC was normal and then 4 months later was LGSIL and testing negative 2 times for HPV but now LGSIL with HPV changes.*

*My doctor also feels my immune system was compromised last year due to the heavy bleeding and anemia. I wonder if taking the BCP can be causing more harm than good now!*

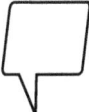

*As someone who has been dealing with this same issue for over two years, I would go straight to the LEEP. This is just my opinion. The reason I say this is because 1. you are done having kinds and 2. your age, although it wouldn't at all be impossible, puts you at more of a disadvantage for clearing the HPV/abnormal cells without medical intervention.*

*I'm 32 and my Pap smears were coming back as HPV+ and ASCUS as well as ASC-H (which is more worrisome than ASCUS) for two years. I had one colposcopy done in May of last year that came back as LGSIL. I had another colposcopy last month that came back HSIL and just had my LEEP four weeks ago where the doctor removed four areas of CIN III. I was much closer to having cervical cancer than I had ever anticipated.*

*If I knew two years ago what I know now, I would have pushed harder for a LEEP right off the bat which would have saved me a LOT of worry, some money, as well as the discomfort and anxiety associated with the subsequent colposcopies needed in order to "monitor" the situation.*

*Of course, with me only being 32 and having no children, it would have been a battle to get a doctor to agree to treat CIN I with a LEEP, but since it came back as CIN III last time, that wasn't an issue.*

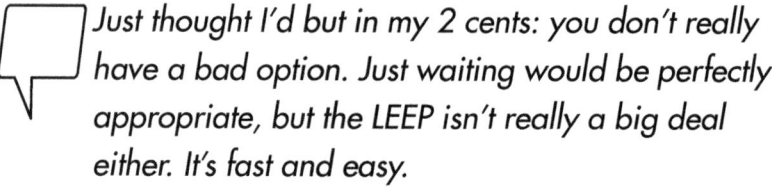

*Just thought I'd but in my 2 cents: you don't really have a bad option. Just waiting would be perfectly appropriate, but the LEEP isn't really a big deal either. It's fast and easy.*

*The pros of the LEEP would be that you're removing the bad cells, and they will have a sample to biopsy to make absolutely sure there is nothing else going on. The cons would be that it is surgery. There is some discomfort (though it's very mild) and there's always a small chance of complications like bleeding. That is really rare with LEEP, because the wire cauterizes at it cuts.*

*With waiting, you could avoid having surgery. Your dysplasia will probably clear up on its own. (It does 70% of the time.) But it could get worse, and then you might have to have a LEEP anyway, and they might have to remove more tissue if your lesions have gotten larger.*

*With either one you probably still have to go in and get checked every few months.*

*I'd probably wait (which is what I did do, until my dysplasia worsened and then I had the LEEP), but if the waiting drives you nuts, have the LEEP. It really is a personal decision in this case since neither one is likely to do you any harm.*

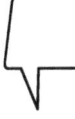

*I agree with others that you really don't have a bad option, just two different ones. Personally, I would go with the LEEP. I've had LSIL and been HPV positive for the past three years and took the wait and see approach. My most recent pap came back as still abnormal but this time couldn't rule out HSIL so my doctor did a LEEP and I thought it was a breeze. The results came back as LSIL but HOPEFULLY that finally cleared out all abnormalities. The reason I'd go straight to the LEEP if it's offered is because 1) it was a lot easier and less painful (for me) than the many*

*colposcopies and biopsies I've had over the past few years and 2) I tend to get really stressed and anxious and have at multiple times felt like I was waiting around for it to get worse rather than better.*

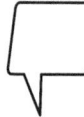

*Were I in your position, I'd opt for treatment immediately. The point of delaying treatment in younger women is to preserve child-carrying potential which is not a consideration at your age. If I didn't care about having children, I would have wanted the HPV and bad cells out of my body yesterday. I'm all for watch and wait as I'm a huge proponent of organic living, healthy eating, supplement taking (where appropriate), holistic healing, etc... but none of this worked for me where HPV of the cervix was concerned. Two years I waited and underwent numerous colposcopies and biopsies and repeat Pap smears and took massive doses of vitamins and stuffed mega doses of vitamins into my vagina in a herculean attempt to remove my HPV and bad cells, until my problem suddenly became much more extensive. At that point, two-year mark, I'd had enough. I had laser and I am glad I did and I hope I don't have to have another but if I do, I will.*

# HPV: THE HUMAN PAPILLOMAVIRUS

*By the way, LEEP is OK, but I'd choose laser over LEEP to reduce (but not eliminate) the chance of stenosis especially in a woman your age; especially if your problems are only on the ectocervix, not endocervix.*

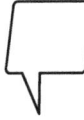

*HPV changes means the presence of koilocytes, which are characteristic of HPV infection and nothing else. Cells have halos and hollow, enlarged and/or multiple nuclei, which is a hallmark of HPV infection.*

*Stenosis can result from any treatment of the cervix, whether LEEP, cone, laser, cryo, cold coagulation, or other. It means the os (opening) of the cervix has closed making future screening difficult or impossible. The gynecologist would dilate your cervix to take a sample. Not the best situation. Laser has a lower incidence of stenosis than the other types of treatment but it is by no means zero.*

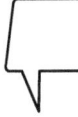

*Speak to your doctor about this, but I think the ECC may have been a false positive.*

*ECCs actually have a high false positive rate when there is dysplasia present on the outside of the cervix. What happens is that some dysplasia from the outside of the cervix contaminates the sample as the curette passes through the opening of your cervix. It totally makes sense if you think about it.*

*With the ECC, what they are really checking for is glandular changes which occur higher up in the cervical canal. Since your ECC did not show glandular changes, and only showed CIN 1, which you have on the outside of your cervix, I would think there is good reason to believe there isn't actually anything going on higher in the canal, and that it was a false positive.*

*With birth control it seems that some studies suggest that it does slightly raise your risk of cervical issues with long term use.*

*After my cone biopsy (a more invasive procedure than what you just had done) I could literally feel the pressure \*down there\* when I was sitting, and found it mildly uncomfortable. It was relieved by lying down, or at least staying semi-reclined, as it took off the pressure. That and some ibuprofen/Motrin will hopefully help!*

*I hadn't realized what he was doing had a name. He just said he was scraping for a good sample, and then off he went... it may explain why the* pain is separate from the stabbing pain where that biopsy that hurt was.

What does it feel like when having an ECC? I heard the biopsy feels like sharp pinch.

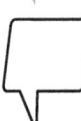

If you've never had menstrual cramps, then the best way I can describe what it felt like (for me) is a Charlie Horse (cramp in the calf). The cramp lasted for about 15–20 seconds, max. After that, I had a dull sensation, similar to a mild stomach ache, for the rest of the day.

Honestly. I'd have an ECC again if it means catching my cancer as early as my ECC helped catch mine. If my doctor hadn't done the ECC, then I'd still have cancer in my cervix and it would still be spreading. Because of the ECC, I am now 11 months cancer free and am looking at going back to annual pelvic exams. I didn't need any chemo or any radiation.

So, bottom line, if a pinch that lasts a few seconds and cramping that lasts a day or so is to be compared with later stages of cancer. That cramping can help detect problems before they become invasive.

 *What is the timeline for being able to have sex prior to having the colposcopy procedure?*

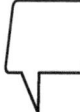 The instructions for preparation for a colposcopy, you aren't to have sex for 24–48 hours before the test or insert anything (tampon, spermicide, etc.) into the vagina as doing so can affect the results of any biopsy you might have. You may want to discuss this with your doctor, just to clarify what he or she wants you to do.

## HISTORY OF VACCINE

In work that was initiated in the mid 1980s, the vaccine was developed, in parallel, by researchers at Georgetown University Medical Center, the University of Rochester, the University of Queensland in Australia, and the U.S. National Cancer Institute.[18] In 2006, the U.S. Food and Drug Administration approved the first preventive HPV vaccine, marketed by Merck & Co. under the trade name Gardasil. According to a Merck press release,[19] in the second quarter 2007, it had been approved in 80 countries, many under fast-track or expedited review. Early in 2007, GlaxoSmithKline filed for approval in the United States for a similar preventive HPV vaccine, known as Cervarix. In June 2007 this vaccine was licensed in Australia, and it was approved in the European Union in September 2007.[20]

### Therapeutic HPV Vaccines

In addition to preventive vaccines, such as Gardasil and Cervarix, laboratory research and several human clinical trials are focused on the development of therapeutic HPV vaccines. In general these vaccines focus on the main HPV oncogenes, E6 and E7. Since expression of E6 and E7 is required for promoting the growth of cervical cancer cells (and cells within warts), it is hoped that immune responses against the two oncogenes might eradicate established tumors.[21]

# HPV: THE HUMAN PAPILLOMAVIRUS

# EPIDEMIOLOGY

## Cutaneous HPVs

Infection with cutaneous HPVs is ubiquitous.[64] Some HPV types, such as HPV-5, may establish infections that persist for the lifetime of the individual without ever manifesting any clinical symptoms. Like remora suckerfish that hitchhike harmlessly on sharks, these HPV types can be thought of as human commensals. Other cutaneous HPVs, such as HPV types 1 or 2, may cause common warts in some infected individuals. Skin warts are most common in childhood and typically appear and regress spontaneously over the course of weeks to months. About 10% of adults also suffer from recurring skin warts. All HPVs are believed to be capable of establishing long-term "latent" infections in small numbers of stem cells present in the skin. Although these latent infections may never be fully eradicated, immunological control is thought to block the appearance of symptoms such as warts. Immunological control is likely HPV type-specific, meaning that an individual may become immunologically resistant to one HPV type while remaining susceptible to other types.

## Genital HPVs

A large increase in the incidence of genital HPV infection occurs at the age when individuals begin to engage in sexual activity. The great majority of genital HPV infections never cause any overt symptoms and are cleared by the immune system in a matter of months. As with cutaneous HPVs, immunity is believed to be HPV type-specific. Some infected individuals may fail to bring genital HPV infection under immunological control. Lingering infection with high-risk HPV types, such as HPVs 16, 18, 31 and 45, can lead to the development of cervical cancer or other types of cancer.[65] In addition to persistent infection with high-risk HPV types, epidemiological and molecular data suggest that co-factors such as the cigarette smoke carcinogen benzo[a]pyrene (BaP) enhance development of certain HPV-induced cancers.[66]

High-risk HPV types 16 and 18 are together responsible for over 65% of cervical cancer cases.[67][6] Type 16 causes 41 to 54% of cervical cancers,[68][6] and accounts for an even greater majority of HPV-induced vaginal/vulvar cancers,[69] penile cancers, anal cancers and head and neck cancers.[70]

# HPV: THE HUMAN PAPILLOMAVIRUS

## PERINATAL TRANSMISSION

Although genital HPV types are sometimes transmitted from mother to child during birth, the appearance of genital HPV-related diseases in newborns is rare. Perinatal transmission of HPV types 6 and 11 can result in the development of juvenile-onset recurrent respiratory papillomatosis (JORRP). JORRP is very rare, with rates of about 2 cases per 100,000 children in the United States.[23] Although JORRP rates are substantially higher if a woman presents with genital warts at the time of giving birth, the risk of JORRP in such cases is still less than 1%.

*Does HPV affect pregnancy or childbirth in ANY way?*

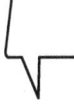

*Generally, no. There's a very, very rare complication of the airways that can occur in babies, but it's happens so rarely that doctors don't even really consider it. A woman with HPV is not expected to have any problems with pregnancy or delivery.*

**HEALTH**SCOUTER

# HPV: THE HUMAN PAPILLOMAVIRUS

## HISTORY OF DISCOVERING A LINK BETWEEN HPV AND CANCER

The fact that prostitutes have much higher rates of cervical cancer than nuns was a key early observation leading researchers to speculate about a causal link between sexually transmitted HPVs and cervical cancer.[71]

Dr. Harald zur Hausen of the German Cancer Research Centre, Heidelberg, Germany, was awarded 2008 Nobel Prize in Physiology or Medicine for his discovery of human papilloma viruses causing cervical cancer.[72] He was interviewed as part of a radio program (HPV - The Shy Virus) about the biology of HPV and the history of the discovery of its connection to cervical cancer.[73]

*If I have genital warts does that make me more likely to get cervical cancer?*

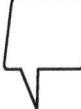

*No, because the types of HPV that cause genital warts are different from the types that cause cervical cancer. However, you can have both kinds at the same time, so you should definitely get yearly gynecological exams.*

*I had a colposcopy today and I was confused about what the doctor was saying. I thought*

*they were checking for cervical cancer and she mentioned that the male passes on HPV to the woman so does that mean that my boyfriend has passed it on to me threw another person or does it mean that it only comes from men in their genes… I don't understand it.*

What she meant is that males often pass on HPV because they are less likely to have symptoms (such as warts). Without symptoms many males do not know they carry the virus and so they unknowingly pass it on. HPV is passed through skin to skin contact and your boyfriend got from someone else, it is not genetic.

HPV is caused by a virus that lives in the skin. It is transmitted by skin to skin contact. The colposcopy was done (probably) because of an abnormal pap result. The pap is a screening test, the colposcopy looks closer to see more specifically at what the outer cervix looks like and better guides the doctor as to what to biopsy. So in that sense, the doctor is (kind of) looking for cellular changes which could lead to cervical cancer.

Something like 99.9% of cervical cancer is caused by HPV.

# HPV: THE HUMAN PAPILLOMAVIRUS

*HPV is not gender specific. Men and women can be infected with HPV: high risk and/or low risk. Most people do not suffer negative effects from HPV. Some do. This is what your doctor was looking for when he/she did the colposcopy.*

*Most people do not know they have HPV (even one or many strains). For that reason, if a person has more than one sexual partner in his/her lifetime, it is very likely he/she has contracted at least one strain of HPV. Because most people do not know they have HPV, if they change partners, then they are spreading any strain of HPV he/she might have, as well as being exposed to (possibly) new strains.*

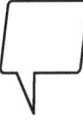

*Your doctor should have said a 'partner' passes on the virus. It is not in men's genes, it's on their skin, and they got it from their past partners, just like it's not in women's genes when they pass it on to their partners.*

*And yes, it is possible to carry the virus for a while before it becomes noticeable with a Pap test.*

*Can a low risk HPV causing genital warts cause penile cancer?*

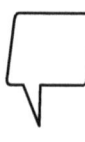 *From what I understand low risk HPV (which causes genital warts) does not lead to cancer. Cancer is caused by high risk HPV which is not detected and/or treated.*

# HPV: THE HUMAN PAPILLOMAVIRUS

# REFERENCES – HPV

1. "STD Facts - Human papillomavirus (HPV)". www.cdc.gov. http://www.cdc.gov/std/HPV/STDFact-HPV.htm. Retrieved on 2009-04-13.

2. Walboomers JM, Jacobs MV, Manos MM, et al (1999). "Human papillomavirus is a necessary cause of invasive cervical cancer worldwide". *J. Pathol.* **189** (1): 12–9. doi:10.1002/(SICI)1096-9896(199909)189:1<12::AID-PATH431>3.0.CO;2-F. PMID 10451482.

3. "NCCC National Cervical Cancer Coalition". http://www.nccc-online.org/. Retrieved on 2008-07-01.

4. Lowy DR, Schiller JT (2006). "Prophylactic human papillomavirus vaccines". *J. Clin. Invest.* **116** (5): 1167–73. doi:10.1172/JCI28607. PMID 16670757.

5. unne EF, Unger ER, Sternberg M, et al (2007). "Prevalence of HPV infection among females in the United States". *JAMA* **297** (8): 813–9. doi:10.1001/jama.297.8.813. PMID 17327523.

6. Baseman JG, Koutsky LA (2005). "The epidemiology of human papillomavirus infections". *J. Clin. Virol.* **32 Suppl 1**: S16–24. doi:10.1016/j.jcv.2004.12.008. PMID 15753008. *Note: The authors state on page S17 "Overall, these DNA-based studies, combined with measurements of type-specific antibodies against HPV capsid antigens, have shown that most (>50%) sexually active women have been infected by one or more genital HPV types at some point in time."

7. "American Social Health Association - HPV Resource Center". http://www.ashastd.org/HPV/HPV_learn_men.cfm. Retrieved on 2007-08-17.

8. "American Social Health Association - National HPV and Cervical Cancer Prevention Resource Center". http://www.ashastd.org/HPV/HPV_learn_patfactsheet.cfm. Retrieved on 2008-07-01.

9. Planned Parenthood "In fact, the lifetime risk for contracting HPV is at least 50 percent for all sexually active women and men, and, it is estimated that, by the age of 50, at least 80 percent of women will have acquired sexually transmitted HPV (CDC, 2004; CDC, 2006)."

10. Medical News Today

11. Dunne EF, Unger ER, Sternberg M, et al (February 2007). "Prevalence of HPV infection among females in the United States". *JAMA : the journal of the American Medical Association* **297** (8): 813–9. doi:10.1001/jama.297.8.813. PMID 17327523.

12. Hillard Weinstock, Stuart Berman and Willard Cates, Jr. (January/February 2004). "Sexually Transmitted Diseases Among American Youth: Incidence and Prevalence Estimates, 2000". *Perspectives on Sexual and Reproductive Health* **36** (1): 6. doi:10.1363/3600604. http://www.guttmacher.org/pubs/journals/3600604.html.

13. Revzina NV, Diclemente RJ (2005). "Prevalence and incidence of human papillomavirus infection in women in the USA: a systematic review". *International journal of STD & AIDS* **16** (8): 528–37. doi:10.1258/0956462054679 214. PMID 16105186."The prevalence of HPV reported in the assessed studies ranged from 14% to more than 90%."

14. McCullough, Marie (2007-02-28). "Cancer-virus strains rarer than first estimated". The Philadelphia Inquirer. http://www.philly.com/mld/inquirer/living/health/16798039.htm. Retrieved on 2007-03-02.

15. Brown, David (2007-02-28). "Study finds more women than expected have HPV". San Francisco Chronicle. http://sfgate.com/cgi-bin/article.cgi?f=/c/a/2007/02/28/MNGOCOCAF61.DTL. Retrieved on 2007-03-02. (originally published in the Washington Post as "More American Women Have HPV Than Previously Thought")

16. Lindsey Tanner (March 11, 2008). "Study Finds 1 in 4 US Teens Has a STD". Newsvine. http://www.newsvine.com/_news/2008/03/11/1358811-study-finds-1-in-4-us-teens-has-a-std. Retrieved on 2008-03-17.

17. "Pap Smear". http://www.imaginis.com/womenshealth/pap_smear.asp. Retrieved on 2008-10-09.

18. "ACS:What Are the Key Statistics About Cervical Cancer?". http://www.cancer.org/docroot/CRI/content/CRI_2_4_1X_What_are_the_key_statistics_for_cervical_cancer_8.asp. Retrieved on 2008-07-01.

19. Bryan JT, Brown DR. Transmission of human papillomavirus type 11 infection by desquamated cornified cells. Virology 2000;281:35-42.

20. Parkin DM (2006). "The global health burden of infection-associated cancers in the year 2002". *Int. J. Cancer* **118** (12): 3030–44. doi:10.1002/ijc.21731. PMID 16404738.

21. a b D'Souza G, Kreimer AR, Viscidi R, *et al* (2007). "Case-control study of human papillomavirus and oropharyngeal cancer". *N. Engl. J. Med.* **356** (19): 1944–56. doi:10.1056/NEJMoa065497. PMID 17494927. http://content.nejm.org/cgi/content/full/356/19/1944.

22. Greenblatt R.J. 2005. Human papillomaviruses: Diseases, diagnosis, and a possible vaccine. *Clinical Microbiology Newsletter,* 27(18), 139–145. Abstract available.

23. Sinal SH, Woods CR (2005). "Human papillomavirus infections of the genital and respiratory tracts in young children". *Seminars in pediatric infectious diseases* **16** (4): 306–16. doi:10.1053/j.spid.2005.06.010. PMID 16210110.

24. Gillison ML, Koch WM, Capone RB, *et al* (2000). "Evidence for a causal association between human papillomavirus and a subset of head and neck cancers". *J. Natl. Cancer Inst.* **92** (9): 709–20. doi:10.1093/jnci/92.9.709. PMID 10793107.

25. Gillison ML (2006). "Human papillomavirus and prognosis of oropharyngeal squamous cell carcinoma: implications for clinical research in head and neck cancers". *J. Clin. Oncol.* **24** (36): 5623–5. doi:10.1200/JCO.2006.07.1829. PMID 17179099.
26. "STD Facts - HPV and Men". http://www.cdc.gov/std/HPV/STDFact-HPV-and-men.htm. Retrieved on 2007-08-17.
27. Frisch M, Smith E, Grulich A, Johansen C (2003). "Cancer in a population-based cohort of men and women in registered homosexual partnerships". *Am. J. Epidemiol.* **157** (11): 966–72. doi:10.1093/aje/kwg067. PMID 12777359. http://171.66.121.65/cgi/content/full/157/11/966. "However, the risk for invasive anal squamous carcinoma, which is believed to be caused by certain types of sexually transmitted human papillomaviruses, notably type 16, was significantly 31-fold elevated at a crude incidence of 25.6 per 100,000 person-years.".
28. Chin-Hong PV, Vittinghoff E, Cranston RD, et al (2005). "Age-related prevalence of anal cancer precursors in homosexual men: the EXPLORE study". *J. Natl. Cancer Inst.* **97** (12): 896–905. doi:10.1093/jnci/dji163. PMID 15956651.
29. http://www.aidsmeds.com/articles/aids_anal_pap_2042_14727.shtml
30. Goldie SJ, Kuntz KM, Weinstein MC, et al. Cost-effectiveness of screening for anal squamous intraepithelial lesions and anal cancer in HIV-negative homosexual and bisexual men. *Amer J of Med* **108:** 634-641, 2000.
31. Mayo Clinic.com, Common warts, http://www.mayoclinic.com/print/common-warts/DS00370/DSECTION=all&METHOD=print
32. Lountzis NI, Rahman O (2008). "Images in clinical medicine. Digital verrucae". *N. Engl. J. Med.* **359** (2): 177. doi:10.1056/NEJMicm071912. PMID 18614785. http://content.nejm.org/cgi/pmidlookup?view=short&pmid=18614785&promo=ONFLNS19.
33. MedlinePlus, Warts, http://www.nlm.nih.gov/medlineplus/warts.html#cat42 (general reference with links). Also, see
34. Greer CE, Wheeler CM, Ladner MB, et al (1995). "Human papillomavirus (HPV) type distribution and serological response to HPV type 6 virus-like particles in patients with genital warts". *J. Clin. Microbiol.* **33** (8): 2058–63. PMID 7559948.
35. Gearheart PA, Randall TC, Buckley RM Jr (2004). "Human Papillomavirus". eMedicine. http://www.emedicine.com/med/topic1037.htm.
36. "STD Facts - Human papillomavirus (HPV)". http://www.cdc.gov/std/HPV/STDFact-HPV.htm. Retrieved on 2007-08-17.
37. http://www.ashastd.org/learn/learn_HPV_warts.cfm
38. http://www.voicemedicine.com/papilloma.htm Photos of larynx Papillomas - Voice Medicine, New York

39. Wu R, Sun S, Steinberg BM (2003). "Requirement of STAT3 activation for differentiation of mucosal stratified squamous epithelium". *Mol. Med.* **9** (3-4): 77–84. doi:10.2119/2003-00001.Wu. PMID 12865943.

40. Moore CE, Wiatrak BJ, McClatchey KD, et al (1999). "High-risk human papillomavirus types and squamous cell carcinoma in patients with respiratory papillomas". *Otolaryngology--head and neck surgery : official journal of American Academy of Otolaryngology-Head and Neck Surgery* **120** (5): 698–705. doi:10.1053/hn.1999.v120.a91773. PMID 10229596.

41. Moore, M. "Tree man 'who grew roots' may be cured" (November 21, 2007). *The Telegraph*.

42. "STD Facts - HPV Vaccine". 2006-08-01. http://www.cdc.gov/std/HPV/STDFact-HPV-vaccine.htm. Retrieved on 2007-08-17.

43. "Pap smears cause cytokine response that may help clear HPV". *OncoLink*. http://www.oncolink.com/resources/article.cfm?c=3&s=8&ss=23&Year=2007&Month=5&id=14201. "J Inflamm 2007;4."

44. Mayrand MH, Duarte-Franco E, Rodrigues I, et al (2007). "Human papillomavirus DNA versus Papanicolaou screening tests for cervical cancer". *N. Engl. J. Med.* **357** (16): 1579–88. doi:10.1056/NEJMoa071430. PMID 17942871. http://content.nejm.org/cgi/pmidlookup?view=short&pmid=17942871&promo=ONFLNS19.

45. Wentzensen, N. and M. von Knebel Doeberitz, Biomarkers in cervical cancer screening. Dis Markers, 2007. 23(4): p. 315-30.

46. Dunne EF, Nielson CM, Stone KM, Markowitz LE, Giuliano AR (2006). "Prevalence of HPV infection among men: A systematic review of the literature". *J. Infect. Dis.* **194** (8): 1044–57. doi:10.1086/507432. PMID 16991079.

47. "Human Papillomavirus (HPV) and Men: Questions and Answers". 2007. http://www.phac-aspc.gc.ca/std-mts/HPV-vph/HPV-vph-man-eng.php. Retrieved on 2008-09-10. "Currently, in Canada there is an HPV DNA test approved for women but not for men."

48. "What Men Need to Know About HPV". 2006. http://www.theHPVtest.com/HPV-for-men-FAQ.html#testmen. Retrieved on 2007-04-04. "There is currently no FDA-approved test to detect HPV in men. That is because an effective, reliable way to collect a sample of male genital skin cells, which would allow detection of HPV, has yet to be developed."

49. Harper DM, Franco EL, Wheeler CM, et al (2006). "Sustained efficacy up to 4.5 years of a bivalent L1 virus-like particle vaccine against human papillomavirus types 16 and 18: follow-up from a randomised control trial". *Lancet* **367** (9518): 1247–55. doi:10.1016/S0140-6736(06)68439-0. PMID 16631880.

50. "Cervarix Package Leaflet: Information for the User". http://emc.medicines.org.uk/emc/assets/c/html/displaydoc.asp?documentid=20207. Retrieved on 2008-06-21.

51. "HPV and HPV Vaccine - HCP". 2006-08-01. http://www.cdc.gov/std/HPV/STDFact-HPV-vaccine-hcp.htm. Retrieved on 2007-08-17.

52. "Centers for Disease Control, HPV Vaccine - Questions & Answers For The Public About the Safety and Effectiveness of the Human Papillomavirus (HPV) Vaccine". http://www.cdc.gov/vaccines/vpd-vac/HPV/HPV-vacsafe-effic.htm. Retrieved on 2007-06-28.

53. "Quadrivalent Human Papillomavirus Vaccine, Recommendations of the Advisory Committee on Immunization Practices" (PDF). *CDC, Morbidity and Mortality Weekly Report Recommendations* **56 / RR-2:** 17, Cervical Cancer Screening Among Vaccinated Females. March 23, 2007. http://www.cdc.gov/mmwr/PDF/rr/rr5602.pdf.

54. "HPV Virus: Information About Human Papillomavirus". WebMD. http://www.webmd.com/sexual-conditions/HPV-genital-warts/HPV-virus-information-about-human-papillomavirus.

55. Vaccination to prevent and treat cervical cancer Hum Pathol. 2004 Aug;35(8):971

56. Markus J. Steiner and Willard Cates, Jr. (2006). "Condoms and Sexually-Transmitted Infections". *N. Engl. J. Med.* **354** (25): 2642–3. doi:10.1056/NEJMp068111. PMID 16790696.[1]

57. Winer RL, Hughes JP, Feng Q, et al (2006). "Condom use and the risk of genital human papillomavirus infection in young women". *N. Engl. J. Med.* **354** (25): 2645–54. doi:10.1056/NEJMoa053284. PMID 16790697.[Free online]

58. Moscicki AB (2005). "Impact of HPV infection in adolescent populations". *The Journal of adolescent health : official publication of the Society for Adolescent Medicine* **37** (6 Suppl): S3–9. PMID 16310138.

59. Bleeker MC, Berkhof J, Hogewoning CJ, et al (2005). "HPV type concordance in sexual couples determines the effect of condoms on regression of flat penile lesions". *Br. J. Cancer* **92** (8): 1388–92. doi:10.1038/sj.bjc.6602524. PMID 15812547.

60. "Planned Parenthood - HPV". http://www.plannedparenthood.org/sexual-health/std/HPV.htm. Retrieved on 2007-08-17.

61. Howett MK, Kuhl JP (2005). "Microbicides for prevention of transmission of sexually transmitted diseases". *Curr. Pharm. Des.* **11** (29): 3731–46. doi:10.2174/138161205774580633. PMID 16305508.

62. Buck CB, Thompson CD, Roberts JN, Müller M, Lowy DR, Schiller JT (2006). "Carrageenan is a potent inhibitor of papillomavirus infection". *PLoS Pathog.* **2** (7): e69. doi:10.1371/journal.ppat.0020069. PMID 16839203.

63. American Cancer Society. "What Are the Risk Factors for Cervical Cancer?". http://www.cancer.org/docroot/CRI/content/CRI_2_4_2X_What_are_the_risk_factors_for_cervical_cancer_8.asp. Retrieved on 2008-02-21.

64. Antonsson A, Forslund O, Ekberg H, Sterner G, Hansson BG (2000). "The ubiquity and impressive genomic diversity of human skin papillomaviruses suggest a commensalic nature of these viruses". *J. Virol.* **74** (24): 11636–41. doi:10.1128/JVI.74.24.11636-11641.2000. PMID 11090162.

65. Schiffman M, Castle PE (2005). "The promise of global cervical-cancer prevention". *N. Engl. J. Med.* **353** (20): 2101–4. doi:10.1056/NEJMp058171. PMID 16291978.

66. Alam S, Conway MJ, Chen HS, Meyers C (2007). "Cigarette Smoke Carcinogen Benzo[a]pyrene Enhances Human Papillomavirus Synthesis". *J Virol* **82**: 1053. doi:10.1128/JVI.01813-07. PMID 17989183.

67. Cohen J (2005). "Public health. High hopes and dilemmas for a cervical cancer vaccine". *Science* **308** (5722): 618–21. doi:10.1126/science.308.5722.618. PMID 15860602.

68. Noel J, Lespagnard L, Fayt I, Verhest A, Dargent J (2001). "Evidence of human papilloma virus infection but lack of Epstein-Barr virus in lymphoepithelioma-like carcinoma of uterine cervix: report of two cases and review of the literature". *Hum. Pathol.* **32** (1): 135–8. doi:10.1053/hupa.2001.20901. PMID 11172309.

69. Edwards QT, Saunders-Goldson S, Morgan PD, Maradiegue A, Macri C (2005). "Vulvar intraepithelial neoplasia: varied signs, varied symptoms: what you need to know". *Advance for nurse practitioners* **13** (3): 49–52. PMID 15777042.

70. Bolt J, Vo QN, Kim WJ, McWhorter AJ, Thomson J, Hagensee ME, Friedlander P, Brown KD, Gilbert J (2005). "The ATM/p53 pathway is commonly targeted for inactivation in squamous cell carcinoma of the head and neck (SCCHN) by multiple molecular mechanisms". *Oral Oncol.* **41** (10): 1013–20. doi:10.1016/j.oraloncology.2005.06.003. PMID 16139561.

71. zur Hausen H, de Villiers EM (1994). "Human papillomaviruses". *Annu. Rev. Microbiol.* **48**: 427–47. doi:10.1146/annurev.micro.48.1.427. PMID 7826013.

72. http://nobelprize.org/nobel_prizes/medicine/laureates/2008/

73. "HPV - the Shy Virus". Soundprint.org radio program. 2008-12-06. http://soundprint.org/radio/display_show/ID/774/name/HPV+-+the+Shy+Virus. Retrieved on 2008-12-06.

## REFERENCES – HPV VACCINE

1. CDC (2006). "STD Facts - HPV Vaccine". http://www.cdc.gov/std/HPV/STDFact-HPV-vaccine.htm. Retrieved on 2007-08-22.

2. Cortez, Michelle Fay and Pettypiece, Shannon. "Merck Cancer Shot Cuts Genital Warts, Lesions in Men". *Bloomberg News*. (Bloomberg.com) 13 Nov 2008.

3. "FDA Approves Expanded Uses for Gardasil to Include Preventing Certain Vulvar and Vaginal Cancers". 2008-09-12. http://www.fda.gov/bbs/topics/NEWS/2008/NEW01885.html. Retrieved on 2008-10-12.

4. Glaxo cervical cancer shot approved in Australia Reuters (2007-05-21) Retrieved on 2007-05-25

5. Jacobs Institute for Women's Health New Report Examines Laws that Would Mandate HPV Vaccine for Young Women

6. Human Papilloma Virus – Common but with dire potential consequences

7. Planned Parenthood "In fact, the lifetime risk for contracting HPV is at least 50 percent for all sexually active women and men, and, it is estimated that, by the age of 50, at least 80 percent of women will have acquired sexually transmitted HPV (CDC, 2004; CDC, 2006)."

8. Medical News Today

9. Dunne EF, Unger ER, Sternberg M, et al. (February 2007). "Prevalence of HPV infection among females in the United States". *JAMA: the journal of the American Medical Association* **297** (8): 813–19. doi:10.1001/jama.297.8.813. PMID 17327523.

10. American Social Health Association "Genital HPV is the most common STD in America; an estimated 80% of sexually active individuals will contract it at some point in their lives."

11. "Study Reveals High Infection Rate In Teens For Virus Linked To Cervical Cancer" Science Daily "The research, reported by Darron R. Brown, M.D., and colleagues at the Indiana University School of Medicine, found four out of five sexually active adolescent females infected with the human papillomavirus."

12. Snijders PJ, Steenbergen RD, Heideman DA, Meijer CJ (2006). "HPV-mediated cervical carcinogenesis: Concepts and clinical implications". *J. Pathol.* **208** (2): 152–64. doi:10.1002/path.1866. PMID 16362994. "cervical cancer is a rare complication of an hrHPV infection since most such infections are transient, not even giving rise to cervical lesions.".

13. "Information from FDA and CDC on Gardasil and its Safety". July 22, 2008. http://www.cdc.gov/vaccinesafety/vaers/FDA_and_CDC_Statement.htm. Retrieved on 2008-08-22.

# HPV: THE HUMAN PAPILLOMAVIRUS

14. Cervical Cancer Action - Funded by the Rockefeller Foundation
15. National Cancer Institute SEER fact sheet on cervical cancer accessed 30 Mar 2007.
16. "Human Papillomavirus (HPV) Vaccines: Q & A - National Cancer Institute". http://www.cancer.gov/cancertopics/factsheet/risk/HPV-vaccine. Retrieved on 2008-07-18.
17. "CDC VAERS - Vaccine Adverse Event Reporting System". http://www.cdc.gov/vaccinesafety/vaers/gardasil.htm. Retrieved on 2009-04-30.
18. McNeil C (April 2006). "Who invented the VLP cervical cancer vaccines?". *Journal of the National Cancer Institute* **98** (7): 433. doi:10.1093/jnci/djj144. PMID 16595773.
19. Merck News Item
20. "Glaxo prepares to launch Cervarix after EU okay". http://www.reuters.com/article/governmentFilingsNews/idUSL2446805720070924. Retrieved on 2008-07-18.
21. Roden RB, Ling M, Wu TC (August 2004). "Vaccination to prevent and treat cervical cancer". *Human pathology* **35** (8): 971–82. doi:10.1016/j.humpath.2004.04.007. PMID 15297964.
22. "HPV Vaccine - Questions & Answers for the Public". http://www.cdc.gov/vaccines/vpd-vac/HPV/HPV-vacsafe-effic.htm. Retrieved on 2008-08-22.
23. National Cancer Institute SEER fact sheet on cervical cancer accessed 30 Mar 2007.
24. "More American Girls And Women Have HPV Than First Thought". http://www.medicalnewstoday.com/articles/64137.php. Retrieved on 2008-05-28.
25. New Report Examines Laws that Would Mandate HPV Vaccine for Young Women George Washington University, December 27, 2007
26. Lowy DR, Schiller JT (May 2006). "Prophylactic human papillomavirus vaccines". *The Journal of clinical investigation* **116** (5): 1167–73. doi:10.1172/JCI28607. PMID 16670757.
27. Women's Health Channel "Cervical Dysplasia: Overview, Risk Factors"]
28. D'Souza G, Kreimer AR, Viscidi R, et al (May 2007). "Case-control study of human papillomavirus and oropharyngeal cancer". The New England journal of medicine 356 (19): 1944–56. doi:10.1056/NEJMoa065497. PMID 17494927.
29. [1]
30. Cottler L, Garvin EC, Callahan C (September 2006). "Condom use and the risk of HPV infection". *The New England journal of medicine* **355** (13): 1388–9; author reply 1389. PMID 17014039.

31. Winer RL, Hughes JP, Feng Q, et al (June 2006). "Condom use and the risk of genital human papillomavirus infection in young women". *The New England journal of medicine* **354** (25): 2645–54. doi:10.1056/NEJMoa053284. PMID 16790697.

32. Baldwin SB, Wallace DR, Papenfuss MR, Abrahamsen M, Vaught LC, Giuliano AR (October 2004). "Condom use and other factors affecting penile human papillomavirus detection in men attending a sexually transmitted disease clinic". *Sexually transmitted diseases* **31** (10): 601–7. PMID 15388997. http://meta.wkhealth.com/pt/pt-core/template-journal/lwwgateway/media/landingpage.htm?issn=0148-5717&volume=31&issue=10&spage=601.

33. Avert.org

34. Genital HPV Infection - CDC Fact Sheet

35. World Health Organization (February 2006). "Fact sheet No. 297: Cancer". http://www.who.int/mediacentre/factsheets/fs297/en/index.html. Retrieved on 2007-12-01.

36. Muñoz N, Bosch FX, Castellsagué X, Díaz M, de Sanjose S, Hammouda D, Shah KV, Meijer CJ (2004-08-20). "Against which human papillomavirus types shall we vaccinate and screen? The international perspective.". *Int J Cancer* **111** (2): 278–85. doi:10.1002/ijc.20244. PMID 15197783.

37. Wittet S. & Tsu V. (2008) Cervical cancer prevention and the Millenium Development Goals. Bulletin of the World Health Organization, 86, 488-490.

38. Cervarix Marketing in Kenya

39. "HPV Vaccine Update". Your Cancer Today. 2007-12-11. http://www.yourcancertoday.com/news/HPV-update.html.

40. 05 Nov 2007, New Data Presented on GARDASIL, Merck's Cervical Cancer Vaccine, in Women Through Age 45. Retrieved through web archive on February 23, 2009

41. Merck Pregnancy Registries - GARDASIL

42. Rosenthal, Elisabeth (2008-08-19). "Drug Makers' Push Leads to Cancer Vaccines' Fast Rise". *The New York Times*. http://www.nytimes.com/2008/08/20/health/policy/20vaccine.html?_r=1&hp=&adxnnl=1&oref=slogin&adxnnlx=1219244494-RoSoOUDyGcwdbs6sjLcrEw. Retrieved on 2008-08-20. "Said Dr. Raffle, the British cervical cancer specialist: "Oh, dear. If we give it to boys, then all pretense of scientific worth and cost analysis goes out the window.""

43. Cancer Research UK. "Gay men seeking HPV vaccine". (http://info.cancerresearch.org). 23 Feb 2007.

44. "Gay men seek 'female cancer' jab". BBC. 2007-02-23. http://news.bbc.co.uk/1/hi/health/6342105.stm.

45. Harper DM, Franco EL, Wheeler CM, et al (April 2006). "Sustained efficacy up to 4.5 years of a bivalent L1 virus-like particle vaccine against human papillomavirus types 16 and 18: follow-up from a randomised control trial". *Lancet* **367** (9518): 1247–55. doi:10.1016/S0140-6736(06)68439-0. PMID 16631880.

46. "FDA Licenses New Vaccine for Prevention of Cervical Cancer and Other Diseases in Females Caused by Human Papillomavirus". FDA. 2006-06-08. http://www.fda.gov/bbs/topics/NEWS/2006/NEW01385.html. Retrieved on 2007-02-04.

47. "New HPV Vaccine Under Study.". Medical College of Georgia, ScienceDaily. 2007-11-20. http://www.sciencedaily.com/releases/2007/11/071119113902.htm. Retrieved on 2008-03-01.

48. Cutts FT, Franceschi S, Goldie S et al. (2007). "Human papillomavirus and HPV vaccines: a review". *Bull World Health Organ* **85** (9): 719–26. doi:10.2471/BLT.06.038414. PMID 18026629. http://www.scielosp.org/scielo.php?script=sci_arttext&pid=S0042-96862007000900018&lng=en&nrm=iso.

49. Australian Government To Fund Cervical Cancer Vaccine Gardasil

50. "Australian Government Funding Of Gardasil". Australian Government Department of Health and Ageing. 2006-11-28. http://www.health.gov.au/internet/main/publishing.nsf/Content/gardasil_HPV.htm. Retrieved on 2008-08-29.

51. Poljak, Vesna; Daley, Gemma (2006-11-29). "Australia to Subsidize Merck Cervical Cancer Vaccine (Update3)". Bloomberg. http://www.bloomberg.com/apps/news?pid=20601081&sid=adOT2d961UKo&refer=australia. Retrieved on 2007-01-26.

52. The Department of Health and Ageing (2007-08-13). "The National HPV Vaccination Program - Frequently Asked Questions for Young Women". http://www.health.gov.au/internet/standby/publishing.nsf/Content/young-women-faq. Retrieved on 2007-09-28.

53. Human Papillomavirus (HPV) Prevention and HPV Vaccine: Questions and Answers

54. HPV Immunization Launched

55. "McGuinty Government Launches Life-Saving HPV Immunization Program:". Premier of Ontario. 2007-08-02. http://www.premier.gov.on.ca/news/Product.asp?ProductID=1552&Lang=EN. Retrieved on 2007-12-02.

56. "HPV Immunization Launched". Province of Nova Scotia. 2007-06-20. http://www.gov.ns.ca/news/details.asp?id=20070620002. Retrieved on 2007-12-02.

57. "British Columbia To Launch Program To Provide HPV Vaccine to Sixth-Grade Girls Next Fall if Approved, Official Says". *Kaiser Daily Women's Health Policy* (Kaiser Family Foundation). 2007-08-09. http://www.kaisernetwork.org/daily_reports/rep_index.cfm?DR_ID=46766. Retrieved on 2007-12-02.

58. "Gardasil authorised for subsidised vaccination". French govt news release (in French). 2007-12-31. http://www.service-public.fr/actualites/00589.html. Retrieved on 2007-12-31.

59. Fagbire, OJ (2007-03-26). "Gardasil, Merck HPV Vaccine, Gets German And Italian Approval For Girls". Vaccine Rx. http://www.vaccinerx.com/news/cervical-cancer/gardasil-merck-HPV-vaccine-gets-german-and-italian-approval-for-girls-20070326-149-26.html. Retrieved on 2007-03-27.

60. fskilkis.gr - T(Pharmacy Association of Kilkis).

61. iaHPV

62. (Romanian) Claudia, Marcu (21 November, 2008) "100.000 de fetițe, injectate cu un vaccin controversat" (100,000 girls injected with a controversial vaccine) Gândul

63. "가다실 제품 허가 공지". 2007-06-27. http://www.msd-korea.com/content/corporate/news/announcement/company22-gardasil.html. Retrieved on 2007-08-06.

64. "Information om det allmänna barnvaccinationsprogrammet" (in Swedish). Smittskyddsinstitutet. http://www.smittskyddsinstitutet.se/hem/mest-efterfragat/allmanna-vaccinationsprogrammet/. Retrieved on 2009-05-06.

65. "NHS Cervical Screening Program". http://www.cancerscreening.nhs.uk/cervical/index.html. Retrieved on 2008-06-26.

66. "1 in 4 US teen girls got cervical cancer shot". http://www.washingtonpost.com/wp-dyn/content/article/2008/10/09/AR2008100901452.html?sub=new. Retrieved on 2008-10-12.

67. HPV Vaccine

68. MIRIAM JORDAN. "Gardasil Requirement for Immigrants Stirs Backlash". The Wall Street Journal. http://online.wsj.com/article/SB122282354408892791.html?. Retrieved on 2009-01-15.

69. HPV Vaccine - Why Your Doctor Doesn't Offer the HPV Vaccine - Gardasil

70. Public Health & Education Detroit News Examines Cost of HPV Vaccine Gardasil - Kaisernetwork.org

71. A question of protection

72. Sprigg, Peter (2006-07-15). "Pro-Family, Pro-Vaccine — But Keep It Voluntary". The Washington Post. http://www.washingtonpost.com/wp-dyn/content/article/2006/07/14/AR2006071401532.html. Retrieved on 2007-02-04.

73. Coyne, Brendan (2005-11-02). "Cervical Cancer Vaccine Raises 'Promiscuity' Controversy". The New Standard. http://newstandardnews.net/content/index.cfm/items/2552. Retrieved on 2006-08-28.

74. Family Research Council: Thursday, February 7, 2008 "IF07B01"

**75.** Focus on the Family Position Statement: Human Papillomavirus Vaccines
**76.** "Lifesaving Politics." Ms. Magazine. pp 12–13. Spring 2007.

# GNU FREE DOCUMENTATION LICENSE

## 0. PREAMBLE

The purpose of this License is to make a manual, textbook, or other functional and useful document "free" in the sense of freedom: to assure everyone the effective freedom to copy and redistribute it, with or without modifying it, either commercially or noncommercially. Secondarily, this License preserves for the author and publisher a way to get credit for their work, while not being considered responsible for modifications made by others.

This License is a kind of "copyleft", which means that derivative works of the document must themselves be free in the same sense. It complements the GNU General Public License, which is a copyleft license designed for free software.

We have designed this License in order to use it for manuals for free software, because free software needs free documentation: a free program should come with manuals providing the same freedoms that the software does. But this License is not limited to software manuals; it can be used for any textual work, regardless of subject matter or whether it is published as a printed book. We recommend this License principally for works whose purpose is instruction or reference.

## 1. APPLICABILITY AND DEFINITIONS

This License applies to any manual or other work, in any medium, that contains a notice placed by the copyright holder saying it can be distributed under the terms of this License. Such a notice grants a world-wide, royalty-free license, unlimited in duration, to use that work under the conditions stated herein. The "Document", herein, refers to any such manual or work. Any member of the public is a licensee, and is addressed as "you". You accept the license if you copy, modify or distribute the work in a way requiring permission under copyright law.

A "Modified Version" of the Document means any work containing the Document or a portion of it, either copied verbatim, or with modifications and/or translated into another language.

A "Secondary Section" is a named appendix or a front-matter section of the Document that deals exclusively with the relationship of the publishers or authors of the Document to the Document's overall subject (or to related matters) and contains nothing that could fall directly within that overall subject. (Thus, if the Document is in part a textbook of mathematics, a Secondary Section may not explain any mathematics.) The relationship could be a matter of historical connection with the subject or with related matters, or of legal, commercial, philosophical, ethical or political position regarding them.

The "Invariant Sections" are certain Secondary Sections whose titles are designated, as being those of Invariant Sections, in the notice that says that the Document is released under this License. If a section does not fit the above definition of Secondary then it is not allowed to be designated as Invariant. The Document may contain zero Invariant Sections. If the Document does not identify any Invariant Sections then there are none.

The "Cover Texts" are certain short passages of text that are listed, as Front-Cover Texts or Back-Cover Texts, in the notice that says that the Document is released under this License. A Front-Cover Text may be at most 5 words, and a Back-Cover Text may be at most 25 words.

A "Transparent" copy of the Document means a machine-readable copy, represented in a format whose specification is available to the general public, that is suitable for revising the document straightforwardly with generic text editors or (for images composed of pixels) generic paint programs or (for drawings) some widely available drawing editor, and that is suitable for input to text formatters or for automatic translation to a variety of formats suitable for input to text formatters. A copy made in an otherwise Transparent file format whose markup, or absence of markup, has been arranged to thwart or discourage subsequent modification by readers is not Transparent. An image format is not Transparent if used for any substantial amount of text. A copy that is not "Transparent" is called "Opaque".

Examples of suitable formats for Transparent copies include plain ASCII without markup, Texinfo input format, LaTeX input format, SGML or XML using a publicly available DTD, and standard-conforming simple HTML, PostScript or PDF designed for human modification. Examples of transparent image formats include PNG, XCF and JPG. Opaque formats include proprietary formats that can be read and edited only by proprietary word processors, SGML or XML for which the DTD and/or processing tools are not generally available, and the machine-generated HTML, PostScript or PDF produced by some word processors for output purposes only.

The "Title Page" means, for a printed book, the title page itself, plus such following pages as are needed to hold, legibly, the material this License requires to appear in the title page. For works in formats which do not have any title page as such, "Title Page" means the text near the most prominent appearance of the work's title, preceding the beginning of the body of the text.

A section "Entitled XYZ" means a named subunit of the Document whose title either is precisely XYZ or contains XYZ in parentheses following text that translates XYZ in another language. (Here XYZ stands for a specific section name mentioned below, such as "Acknowledgements", "Dedications", "Endorsements", or "History".) To "Preserve the Title" of such a section when you modify the Document means that it remains a section"Entitled XYZ" according to this definition.

The Document may include Warranty Disclaimers next to the notice which states that this License applies to the Document. These Warranty Disclaimers are considered to be included by reference in this License, but only as regards disclaiming warranties: any other implication that these Warranty Disclaimers may have is void and has no effect on the meaning of this License.

## 2. VERBATIM COPYING

You may copy and distribute the Document in any medium, either commercially or noncommercially, provided that this License, the copyright notices, and the license notice saying this License applies to the Document are reproduced in all copies, and that you add no other conditions whatsoever to those of this License. You may not use technical measures to obstruct or control the reading or further copying of the copies you make or distribute. However, you may accept compensation in exchange for copies. If you distribute a large enough number of copies you must also follow the conditions in section 3.

You may also lend copies, under the same conditions stated above, and you may publicly display copies.

## 3. COPYING IN QUANTITY

If you publish printed copies (or copies in media that commonly have printed covers) of the Document, numbering more than 100, and the Document's license notice requires Cover Texts, you must enclose the copies in covers that carry, clearly and legibly, all these Cover Texts: Front-Cover Texts on the front cover, and Back-Cover Texts on the back cover. Both covers must also clearly and legibly identify you as the publisher of these copies. The front cover must present the full title with all words of the title equally prominent and visible. You may add other material on the covers in addition. Copying with changes limited to the covers, as long as they preserve the title of the Document and satisfy these conditions, can be treated as verbatim copying in other respects.

If the required texts for either cover are too voluminous to fit legibly, you should put the first ones listed (as many as fit reasonably) on the actual cover, and continue the rest onto adjacent pages.

If you publish or distribute Opaque copies of the Document numbering more than 100, you must either include a machine-readable Transparent copy along with each Opaque copy, or state in or with each Opaque copy a computer-network location from which the general network-using public has access to download using public-standard network protocols a complete Transparent copy of the Document, free of added material. If you use the latter option, you must take reasonably prudent steps, when you begin distribution of Opaque copies in quantity, to ensure that this Transparent copy will remain thus accessible at the stated location until at least one year after the last time you distribute an Opaque copy (directly or through your agents or retailers) of that edition to the public.

It is requested, but not required, that you contact the authors of the Document well before redistributing any large number of copies, to give them a chance to provide you with an updated version of the Document.

## 4. MODIFICATIONS

You may copy and distribute a Modified Version of the Document under the conditions of sections 2 and 3 above, provided that you release the Modified Version under precisely this License, with the Modified Version filling the role of the Document, thus licensing distribution and modification of the Modified Version to whoever possesses a copy of it. In addition, you must do these things in the Modified Version:

- **A.** Use in the Title Page (and on the covers, if any) a title distinct from that of the Document, and from those of previous versions (which should, if there were any, be listed in the History section of the Document). You may use the same title as a previous version if the original publisher of that version gives permission.
- **B.** List on the Title Page, as authors, one or more persons or entities responsible for authorship of the modifications in the Modified Version, together with at least five of the principal authors of the Document (all of its principal authors, if it has fewer than five), unless they release you from this requirement.

C. State on the Title page the name of the publisher of the Modified Version, as the publisher.

D. Preserve all the copyright notices of the Document.

E. Add an appropriate copyright notice for your modifications adjacent to the other copyright notices.

F. Include, immediately after the copyright notices, a license notice giving the public permission to use the Modified Version under the terms of this License, in the form shown in the Addendum below.

G. Preserve in that license notice the full lists of Invariant Sections and required Cover Texts given in the Document's license notice.

H. Include an unaltered copy of this License.

I. Preserve the section Entitled "History", Preserve its Title, and add to it an item stating at least the title, year, new authors, and publisher of the Modified Version as given on the Title Page. If there is no section Entitled "History" in the Document, create one stating the title, year, authors, and publisher of the Document as given on its Title Page, then add an item describing the Modified Version as stated in the previous sentence.

J. Preserve the network location, if any, given in the Document for public access to a Transparent copy of the Document, and likewise the network locations given in the Document for previous versions it was based on. These may be placed in the "History" section. You may omit a network location for a work that was published at least four years before the Document itself, or if the original publisher of the version it refers to gives permission.

K. For any section entitled "Acknowledgements" or "Dedications", Preserve the Title of the section, and preserve in the section all the substance and tone of each of the contributor acknowledgements and/or dedications given therein.

L. Preserve all the Invariant Sections of the Document, unaltered in their text and in their titles. Section numbers or the equivalent are not considered part of the section titles.

M. Delete any section entitled "Endorsements". Such a section may not be included in the Modified Version.

N. Do not retitle any existing section to be entitled "Endorsements" or to conflict in title with any Invariant Section.

O. Preserve any Warranty Disclaimers.

If the Modified Version includes new front-matter sections or appendices that qualify as Secondary Sections and contain no material copied from the Document, you may at your option designate some or all of these sections as Invariant. To do this, add their titles to the list of Invariant Sections in the Modified Version's license notice. These titles must be distinct from any other section titles.

You may add a section entitled "Endorsements", provided it contains nothing but endorsements of your Modified Version by various parties—for example, statements of peer review or that the text has been approved by an organization as the authoritative definition of a standard.

You may add a passage of up to five words as a Front-Cover Text, and a passage of up to 25 words as a Back-Cover Text, to the end of the list of Cover Texts in the Modified Version. Only one passage of Front-Cover Text and one of Back-Cover Text may be added by (or through arrangements made by) any one entity. If the Document already includes a Cover Text for the same cover, previously added by you or by arrangement made by the same entity you are acting on behalf of, you may not add another; but you may replace the old one, on explicit permission from the previous publisher that added the old one.

The author(s) and publisher(s) of the Document do not by this License give permission to use their names for publicity for or to assert or imply endorsement of any Modified Version.

## 5. COMBINING DOCUMENTS

You may combine the Document with other documents released under this License, under the terms defined in section 4 above for modified versions, provided that you include in the combination all of the Invariant Sections of all of the original documents, unmodified, and list them all as Invariant Sections of your combined work in its license notice, and that you preserve all their Warranty Disclaimers.

The combined work need only contain one copy of this License, and multiple identical Invariant Sections may be replaced with a single copy. If there are multiple Invariant Sections with the same name but different contents, make the title of each such section unique by adding at the end of it, in parentheses, the name of the original author or publisher of that section if known, or else a unique number. Make the same adjustment to the section titles in the list of Invariant Sections in the license notice of the combined work.

In the combination, you must combine any sections entitled "History" in the various original documents, forming one section entitled "History";

likewise combine any sections entitled "Acknowledgements", and any sections entitled "Dedications". You must delete all sections entitled "Endorsements."

## 6. COLLECTIONS OF DOCUMENTS

You may make a collection consisting of the Document and other documents released under this License, and replace the individual copies of this License in the various documents with a single copy that is included in the collection, provided that you follow the rules of this License for verbatim copying of each of the documents in all other respects.

You may extract a single document from such a collection, and distribute it individually under this License, provided you insert a copy of this License into the extracted document, and follow this License in all other respects regarding verbatim copying of that document.

## 7. AGGREGATION WITH INDEPENDENT WORKS

A compilation of the Document or its derivatives with other separate and independent documents or works, in or on a volume of a storage or distribution medium, is called an "aggregate" if the copyright resulting from the compilation is not used to limit the legal rights of the compilation's users beyond what the individual works permit. When the Document is included in an aggregate, this License does not apply to the other works in the aggregate which are not themselves derivative works of the Document.

If the Cover Text requirement of section 3 is applicable to these copies of the Document, then if the Document is less than one half of the entire aggregate, the Document's Cover Texts may be placed on covers that bracket the Document within the aggregate, or the electronic equivalent of covers if the Document is in electronic form. Otherwise they must appear on printed covers that bracket the whole aggregate.

## 8. TRANSLATION

Translation is considered a kind of modification, so you may distribute translations of the Document under the terms of section 4. Replacing Invariant Sections with translations requires special permission from their copyright holders, but you may include translations of some or all Invariant Sections in addition to the original versions of these Invariant Sections. You may include a translation of this License, and all the license notices in the Document, and any Warranty Disclaimers, provided that you also include the original English version of this License and the original versions of those notices and disclaimers. In case of a disagreement between the translation and the original version of this License or a notice or disclaimer, the original version will prevail.

If a section in the Document is entitled "Acknowledgements", "Dedications", or "History", the requirement (section 4) to Preserve its Title (section 1) will typically require changing the actual title.

## 9. TERMINATION

You may not copy, modify, sublicense, or distribute the Document except as expressly provided for under this License. Any other attempt to copy, modify, sublicense or distribute the Document is void, and will automatically terminate your rights under this License. However, parties who have received copies, or rights, from you under this License will not have their licenses terminated so long as such parties remain in full compliance.

## 10. FUTURE REVISIONS OF THIS LICENSE

The Free Software Foundation may publish new, revised versions of the GNU Free Documentation License from time to time. Such new versions will be similar in spirit to the present version, but may differ in detail to address new problems or concerns. See http://www.gnu.org/copyleft/.

Each version of the License is given a distinguishing version number. If the Document specifies that a particular numbered version of this License "or any later version" applies to it, you have the option of following the terms and conditions either of that specified version or of any later version that has been published (not as a draft) by the Free Software Foundation. If the Document does not specify a version number of this License, you may choose any version ever published (not as a draft) by the Free Software Foundation.

# INDEX

Anal Sex, 20, 41, 73
ASCUS, 58, 59, 61–63, 92, 101, 104
Cancer, 31, 39, 40, 47, 53, 96, 113, 119, 122
Cancer, Cervical, 15, 31–33, 39, 40, 44, 53, 55, 56, 59–61, 64, 70, 75, 79, 85, 86, 91, 92, 94–96, 100, 105, 113, 116, 119, 120
Cancer Prevention, 53
Carrageenan, 87
Cervarix, 77, 113
Childbirth, 117
Colposcopy, 54, 58, 60–64, 76, 97–102, 105, 112, 119–121
Condoms, 20, 21, 46, 73, 75, 85
Dysplasia, 56, 83, 91, 93–101, 103, 104, 107, 109
ECC, 60, 76, 98, 101, 104, 105, 109–111
Epidemiology, 115
Focal Epithelial Hyperplasia, 37
Gardasil, 16, 26, 45, 46, 77, 79, 80–82, 91, 92, 113
Genital Warts. See Warts
GNU Free Documentation License, 136

HPV, 15–23, 25–29, 31, 32, 35–37, 39–41, 43–47, 49, 51, 53, 55–59, 62, 63, 65–67, 69–83, 85–87, 89, 91–93, 96–98, 100–105, 107–109, 113, 115–117, 119–122
HPV, Associated Diseases, 37
HPV, Cutaneous, 4, 37, 40, 53, 87, 115, 116, 119
HPV, Genital, 116
HPV Infection, 96
HPV Lifecycle, 35
HPV Testing, 69
HPV Testing, Males, 73
HPV Vaccines, 77
Human Papillomavirus. See HPV
Immunocompromised Patients, 51
Infection, Rate of, 25
Introduction, 15
JORRP, 117
Latency Period, 36
LEEP, 61, 63, 93, 101, 103–107, 109
LGSIL, 93
Microbicides, 87
Multivitamin, 66
Neoplasia, 37, 73
Oncogenes, 35, 39, 79, 113

Oral Papillomas, 37
Pap Smear, 15, 19, 41, 54, 55,
    57, 58, 65, 66, 69, 71, 76, 79,
    92, 94, 101, 104
Penis, 17, 28
Perinatal Transmission, 117
Plantar Warts. See Warts
Pregnancy, 117
Prevalence, 25
Respiratory Papillomatosis,
    3, 49
Risk Factors, 96
Seropostive, 80
Stenosis, 109
Strains, 18, 23, 26–28, 32, 39,
    57, 74, 96, 121
Treatment, 89
Vaccination, 77, 78, 91, 92
Vaccine, 91
Vaccine, History Of, 113
Vaccines, Therapeutic, 113
Verrucae. See Warts
Viral Genome, 35
Vitamins, 66, 108
Warts, 15–18, 20, 23, 28, 31,
    32, 37, 43–47, 49, 51, 58, 73,
    74, 77, 79, 82, 86, 91, 96, 103,
    114, 115, 117, 119–122

www.ingramcontent.com/pod-product-compliance
Ingram Content Group UK Ltd.
Pitfield, Milton Keynes, MK11 3LW, UK
UKHW021303180426
11947UKWH00015B/987